FORGET "REMEMBER"

13 Steps to Care

A Guidebook for the Dementia Caregiver

By: Dennis E. Wiseman

About the author

Dennis Wiseman has facilitated the Good Shepherd Support Group for over twenty years. Dennis had to learn about Alzheimer's and dementia the hard way. His mother was diagnosed which left him as the sole caregiver. Married and raising his own family, challenged with a new job, and the primary caregiver for his mother, made it very difficult for Dennis to deal with his own life struggles. He turned to the support group for help. Since, he has studied and has learned a great deal about the disease; he has participated in panel discussions; and was a part of the Alzheimer's Association speaker's bureau. Dennis has developed Forget "Remember" and shares this material as part of his group discussions. He presents this material in a very easy-to-read format. Dennis' intent is to make this book a training guide that all can understand. His style can be witful at times so as to add character and humanize the material at hand. Sometimes that one simple smile that may result from a reading in this book could provide a great deal of healing that the reader was so desperately seeking.

It is Dennis' passion to present this material to the hundreds of thousands of caregivers worldwide that struggle each and every day alongside a loved-one stricken with a life-ending dementia. Until a cure is available, this material should inspire, enlighten, and strengthen you so that you can face another day.

Disclaimer – I am neither a medical doctor or a licensed attorney. Anything in my writings that appears to be medical or legal advice is implied as something for you to consider and then seek professional advice or counsel. Due to the nature of the diseases, the recommendations suggested within may not be effective with your given set of circumstances. With many years of experience in working within the Alzheimer's arena, I have learned some very valuable techniques, thoughts, and considerations that I am sharing with you. Although this book is written in the United States with reference to the US medical and legal systems, I in no way wish to assume nor preclude the use of this material in principle in other countries or providences. All individuals referenced as examples, although factual, have no connection to the actual individual or associated family.

Copyright © 2018 by Dennis E. Wiseman

Available from Amazon.com, CreateSpace.com, and other retail outlets.
First Printing, 2018

ISBN 978-0-692-17008-3

VIGILANT METHODS, LLC.

Table of Contents

This book is presented to you in a three-section format. The first section is designed to provide some preliminary information to help you understand the role of the caregiver. In the second section, I share my 13 Steps to Care. Each of these steps are carefully designed and recommended to you so you can best provide that so important "Quality of Life" to your loved-one. The third section includes several Tips and Tricks I have learned and am now sharing them with you. At the very back of the book you will find a few Notes pages. Please use these pages as you need. I urge you to write all throughout the book, underlining, highlighting, and folding over corners.

This is your Guidebook for the Dementia Caregiver!

SECTION 1

This first section of this book will help you as the caregiver, care provider, family member, friend, relative, or just someone that has decided to obtain a better understanding of dementia, its characteristics, its devastation, and how to manage your way through it. I will explain the term dementia, we will explore the definition of some common words used throughout the book, recognize how every person is unique, see what it takes to be an effective caregiver, and learn some basic rules to follow in order to provide that "Quality of Life" that we all hope to maintain.

In the Beginning...

God created man and called him Adam. Following, God created woman from man and all was good. God said to both, do not eat from the "Tree of Good and Evil." Most know what happened. This was the first documented incident of dementia.

So, let's better understand the term dementia. According to the Alzheimer's Association, they say, *"Dementia is not a specific disease. It's an overall term that describes a group of symptoms associated with a decline in memory or other thinking skills severe enough to reduce a person's ability to perform everyday activities."* The foremost condition is loss of memory or sometimes referred to as Mild Cognitive Impairment. Dementia effects our motor skills to where we may need assistance to

> **Dementia is not a disease; it is a group of symptoms that impact memory.**

perform some of our common life-based activities. Even confusion and disorientation are affected that can extend to an actual behavioral shift. We may hallucinate, become paranoid, and experience delusions. Left untreated, these conditions can continue to worsen. Our brain can self-diagnose itself into an irreversible condition causing us to pull away from family and friends, lose any sexual interests, disrupt our sleep, and find our way into a deeper confusion. None of what has been explained here is a disease. It is your brain snowballing your body to convince you of something that may actually be curable.

When the doctor issues the diagnosis of Alzheimer's, Vascular Dementia, Lewy Bodies, Parkinson's, Pick's, Creutzfeldt-Jakob, and Huntington's, you will hear the one thing common to all of these; they are a disease. It is possible to have more than one. In some cases, one can lead to another, similar to cancer. Each of these various diseases have a unique effect on the brain and all are considered non-curable.

Let's Define Some of the Terms You Will See Used in This Book

These are some terms that will be discussed in this book. To avoid confusion, I thought it would be best that we establish a common definition in advance. Some of these terms may vary slightly when in reference to other illnesses or conditions that do not include dementia care.

Alzheimer's – is a progressive mental deterioration that can occur in middle or old age, due to generalized degeneration of the brain. Symptoms usually develop slowly and get worse over time, becoming severe enough to interfere with daily tasks. It is the most common cause of premature senility. Alzheimer's is considered an unrecoverable disease.

Assisted living facility – is a housing alternative for older adults who may need help with dressing, bathing, eating, and toileting, but do not require the intensive medical and nursing care provided in nursing homes.

Caregiver – is typically a family member, otherwise, a paid helper who provides help to another person. For purposes of this book, the caregiver is the primary person providing the help.

Caregiving – is the act of providing assistance and support to family members or acquaintances who have physical, psychological, or developmental needs. Caring for others generally takes on three forms: instrumental, emotional, and informational caring.

Cognitive impairment - is when a person has trouble remembering, learning new things, concentrating, or making decisions that affect their everyday life. Cognitive impairment ranges from mild to severe. This is typically diagnosed by a medical professional and documented.

Degenerative dementia – is when the dementia continually gets worse causing a noticeable decline in cognitive ability. Much of this book relates to this type of dementia.

Demented – is the suffering from a severe mental illness, especially Alzheimer's disease. An informal definition is when someone is driven to behave irrationally due to anger, distress, or excitement.

Dementia – is a temporary or permanent loss of memory. Dementia is not a disease, but a medical condition or category. It is possible to have more than one type of dementia.

Full care nursing facility – (now known as a Long-Term Care Facility,) is a place for people who do not need to be in a hospital but cannot be cared for at home. Most nursing homes have nursing aides and skilled nurses on hand 24-hours a day. Some nursing homes are set up like a hospital. The staff provides medical care, as well as physical, speech and occupational therapy. In the US, these facilities are typically regulated by their state health department.

General Practitioner (GP) – is a medical doctor with a focus on acute and chronic illnesses. This doctor also provides preventive care and treats patients of all ages and gender. The GP also known as the generalist is considered the "family doctor."

Geriatrician – is a medical doctor who specializes in the diagnosis, treatment, and prevention of disease and disability in older adults. Geriatric physicians are primary care doctors who are specially trained in the aging process.

Loved-one – is a person one loves and especially a member of one's family (or extended family) that is in need of care and becomes dependent upon you to help in providing the various levels of care.

Patient/Victim – is any recipient of health care services. The patient is most often ill or injured and in need of life sustaining assistance.

Psychologist – focus extensively on psychotherapy and treating emotional and mental suffering in patients with behavioral intervention. A psychologist typically cannot write prescriptions.

Psychiatrist – is a licensed medical doctor, they can prescribe medications, and they spend much of their time with patients on medication management as a course of treatment. Often, you will find the psychologist and the psychiatrist working together to treat a patient's symptoms.

Quality of life – is a sense of well-being by obtaining a level of comfort, happiness, wealth, education, and family values. Quality of life becomes a unit of measurement in determining a person's state of euphoria. Quality typically denotes a circle of continuous improvement.

Quantity of life – is your years of existence. How long you have lived and how long you want to live. Quality versus Quantity is sometimes confused. Quantity without Quality can be considered disrespectful to the individual receiving the care.

Therapeutic fibbing – is a controversial yet very effective method of dealing with the anxiety experienced by many people with Alzheimer's and other dementias. For the most part, it is telling a "fib" in order to avoid increased anxiety and agitation in a person with dementia.

Trusted advisor – an individual in which one can place complete trust, in knowing this person is always working to protect, provide, and care for them without self-interest or personal gain. A person with dementia needs an individual that will always be concerned for the quality of life conditions. The trusted advisor is typically the family member closest to the patient.

Validate – is to prove that something is based on truth or fact. You may need someone to validate your feelings or comments in order to allow you to feel accepted or believed.

Ten Warning Signs of Alzheimer's

Reprinted with permission by the Alzheimer's Association®

1. Memory loss - It's normal to occasionally forget an assignment, deadline or colleague's name, but frequent forgetfulness or unexplainable confusion at home or in the workplace may signal that something's wrong.

2. Difficulty performing familiar tasks - Busy people get distracted from time to time. For example, you might leave something on the stove too long or not remember to serve part of a meal. People with Alzheimer's might prepare a meal and not only forget to serve it, but also forget they made it.

3. Problems with language - Everyone has trouble finding the right word sometimes, but a person with Alzheimer's may forget simple words or substitute inappropriate words, making sentences difficult to understand.

4. Disorientation to time and place - It's normal to momentarily forget the day of the week or what you need from the store. But people with Alzheimer's can become lost on their own street, not knowing where they are, how they got there or how to get back home.

5. Poor or decreased judgment - Choosing not to bring a sweater along on a chilly night is a common mistake. A person with Alzheimer's, however, may dress inappropriately in more noticeable ways, wearing a bathrobe to the store or several blouses on a hot day.

6. Problems with abstract thinking - Balancing a checkbook can be challenging for many people, but for someone with Alzheimer's, recognizing numbers or performing basic calculations may be impossible.

7. Misplacing things - Everyone temporarily misplaces a wallet or keys from time to time. A person with Alzheimer's disease may put these and other items in inappropriate places -- such as an iron in the freezer, or a wristwatch in the sugar bowl -- then not recall how they got there.

8. Changes in mood or behavior - Everyone experiences a broad range of emotions – it's part of being human. People with Alzheimer's tend to exhibit more rapid mood swings for no apparent reason.

9. Changes in personality - People's personalities may change somewhat as they age. But a person with Alzheimer's can change dramatically, either suddenly or over a period of time. Someone who is generally easy going may become angry, suspicious or fearful.

10. Loss of initiative - It's normal to tire of housework, business activities, or social obligations, but most people retain or eventually regain their interest. The person with Alzheimer's disease may remain disinterested and uninvolved in many or all of his usual pursuits.

Altimers? Oldtimers? Alheimer?...
No, it is Alzheimer's (älts͵hīmərz)

There are nearly one hundred different types of dementia. They range from the guys night out on the town with far too much to drink and not remembering why in the morning he finds a phone number in his pocket written on a napkin from Bruce and thanking him for the lovely evening; to the irreversible fatal Alzheimer's Disease. Dementias are in two categories, curable and non-curable. Alzheimer's Disease for example is a non-curable, fatal disease. If the disease runs its full course, the

It is estimated by 2020, there will be over 50 million people worldwide living with dementia.

victim will eventually forget to breathe, or the involuntary heartbeat will not process and end the life. So, what are the dementias that have inspired me to write this book? They are Alzheimer 's disease, Vascular disease, Lewy bodies dementia, Picks disease, frontotemporal dementia, HIV-associated dementia, Huntington's disease, Dementia Pugilistica, Corticobasal degeneration, Creutzfeldt-Jakob disease, Multiple Sclerosis, Amyotrophic Lateral Sclerosis (ALS) dementia, Olivopontocerebellar Atrophy (OPCA), Wilson's disease, hydrocephalus, and other rare hereditary dementias. Some of these listed are considered hereditary while others are as of yet not known even to the extent of how or why they develop. Alzheimer's disease and Vascular dementia are the two most common forms of dementia.

This book will reference Alzheimer's disease as a more generic term. Alzheimer's disease is a specific dementia, it shares many of the same characteristics as with most other more common dementias. Since Alzheimer's is the most common form of an irreversible dementia, it is the common theme of this book.

I recently attended an Alzheimer's Memory Walk event in my area held in a beautiful outdoor park with a pavilion, pathways, and large trees. I was sitting on a bench outside the registration area. A bus pulled up from one of the local long-term care facilities. I was not paying close attention to those coming off the bus because I was there to meet some of my fellow group members. A woman came up to me and asked if I would mind her sharing the bench with me. I agreed and smiled. Within a few minutes, I had several people in front of me; both in wheelchairs and standing. One of the care providers positioned a woman just off to my right and asked if she would be in my way. "Of course not," I replied. I turned to the woman next to me; again, not sure if she arrived on the bus and mentioned to her how beautiful the day is. She agreed saying it is a beautiful day. I then asked her why she was here today. She replied, "I guess I am here to help find that woman over there a place to stay." I quickly figured out that indeed, she did recently arrive on the bus.

Everyone is Different

Our planet has about seven quintillion, five hundred quadrillion grains of sand. (At last count of course.) Considering how many grains of sand exist, there are no two exactly alike. To the naked eye, they all look alike, but under magnification, there are miraculous differences. This holds true with snowflakes, tree leaves, and flower blooms. This also applies to humans. Identical twins are no longer "identical" once the first one takes a breath while the other is still exiting the birth canal. From that point forward, although there is a DNA match, they are no longer identical. From that point forward, they continue on a journey of developing their own uniqueness. There comes a time later in life that these unique characteristics will become noticeable. You will never find two people the same. You will never find two Alzheimer's patients that are the same. As with the identical twins, they have been exposed to different foods, various airborne pollutants, an array of cleaning and workplace chemicals, variations in flu-shot strains, and a multitude of cosmetics or fragrances. Each and every component will then react uniquely to the body as a result of all the other exposures. There is an expression used within the Alzheimer's communities that says, "If you know one Alzheimer's patient, then you only know one Alzheimer's patient." This means everyone is different.

I had several family members come to my support group telling me their loved-one was at Stage 11, Stage 2 or Stage 4. When I would ask what scale they were using, I was told it was something their doctor shared or from a chart they saw on the internet. I have seen charts that range from 3-Stages to over 21-Stages. The Alzheimer's Association is currently using the 7-Stage model. In mentioning above how no two dementia patients are alike, so too is their progress through the stages. Some may display signs from Stage 1 and Stage 3 at the same time. So, at what Stage do they reside? I would urge you to not focus on the stages of progression. I assure you, this is no contest you want to win. Simply put your focus on the conditions at hand. As you read through this book, I am hopeful that you will be better prepared when the next stage arrives. Because of the variations of the body's chemistry, some characteristics unique to a specific stage may or may not occur. Wandering is a common trait, but as mentioned, it may become an issue with your loved-one or not. Let's pray for the best.

Estimated timeframes within the primary stages:

Mild, early stage 2 – 4 years
Moderate stage 2 – 10 years
Severe stage 1 – 3 years

Baseline Criteria

Nearly all professional sports players, senior leaders of countries, astronauts, and even high school swim team members have to endure a full mental and physical evaluation prior to playing their sport or fulfilling their professional role. Everything is tested and documented. This is called a baseline comprehensive physical examination and is the foundation where future tests are compared. If the player receives a concussion, in comparing the baseline evaluation, the medical team will be better prepared to take the needed corrective action. Once the player has returned to health and the medical team is comfortable that the player has returned to his normal self, he is released back into play.

This evaluation is also needed for a dementia patient. I am not suggesting it to be as comprehensive, but it would be beneficial to have an extensive examination. I say this for two reasons. First, there are times where medical professionals may miss the diagnosis and treat for the wrong illness. In some cases, this can actually aggravate the condition causing it to worsen. Second, as changes occur and markers are determined, future testing may indicate a course change. Examples of these are when trying to diagnose Alzheimer's disease, it is often the symptoms that determine the diagnosis rather than a conclusive analysis. This is mainly because, there is no 100% conclusive way of diagnosing Alzheimer's disease. This misalignment can cause a delay in treating the actual illness. A complete blood count (CBC) is the most common blood test that is generally advised to evaluate the overall health of an individual and detect/diagnose a wide range of disorders, that include anemia (deficiency of RBC/Hemoglobin), infection and leukemia (Cancer of blood/bone marrow). Over a period of time, if you find the hemoglobin (red blood cells) levels continue to drop, there can be problems with iron, folic acid, and Vitamin B12. As the B12 level drops further, dementia conditions may begin to appear.

In both examples, if you were able to reference the baseline evaluations, you will quickly begin to see a variance that may not get noticed by the medical provider. You will read in this book the importance of a qualified and trusted primary care physician. You will also read where I explain that it is not their sole full-time job to keep your loved-one healthy. You have to be proactive. You need to intervene. You are their advocate.

Caregiving

No one is born a caregiver. Although we can learn how to provide health care services to others, we cannot be taught to be compassionate, empathetic, patient, and a nurturer. These are all personality traits that originate from the heart. In all areas, you must want to be that person. Because you have all or most of these traits is the reason you have decided to be that provider for your loved-one and why you are reading this book. It is not that you do not trust others, it is something deep inside you that makes you personally decide

> **The three most valuable traits of a dementia caregiver: Compassion, Empathy, and Patience.**

this is what you should be doing. If you lack these traits, it may be best to ask for help from others as much as possible. Having personally listened to and studied hundreds of caregiver's stories, I am convinced that you are the caregiver because your loved-one had already secretly chosen you to be that person for them.

When working with those with dementia, often they really do not know what they need. They may not know if they are cold or if their knee is hurting. If the care provider lacks the traits I just mentioned, the patient may be sitting there in a very cold area, while the care provider is getting frustrated because they were told everything is fine. However, we are getting a high level of agitation coming from the patient. Have you been in a hospital bed wishing you had a blanket because the room was so cold? You have already pushed the "nurse call button" and have received no response. You are getting more upset by the minute. There is no one else to ask since you are in your room alone. Finally, your nurse shows up at your door, you bark at her telling her to get you a blanket. In this example, you were able to explain what you need. Your loved-one may not have the ability to effectively communicate his needs. This is why compassion is important. You want to be able to best understand your patient's needs. <u>Compassion</u> motivates people to go out of their way to help the physical, mental, and emotional pains of another. By being <u>empathetic</u>, you are trying to understand what your loved-one is feeling by trying to feel what they are experiencing. In the case of the room temperature, it is stopping for a moment and feeling, seeing, smelling, and listening to the environment to sense what they might be sensing. <u>Patience</u> is not sitting and waiting, it is the ability to remain calm while dealing with a difficult situation. If you display irritation or frustration, your patient will pick up on that and likely react in a similar fashion. A great example is when working with your loved-one to do something needed. They are resisting, and you become frustrated and start raising your voice. This will only cause them to pull back further to the extent of either an all-out screaming match or a tear fest explodes. By staying firm and demonstrating patience, you can approach the task more calmly; think about your wording; speak slower and softer; and lead them, not force them. **Life is giving you this moment; embrace it.** It is up to you to decide how to handle it. A patient, compassionate caregiver will likely produce the better outcome.

> *Caregiving is not an obligation; it is a privilege.*

I recall a story that Margie shared with me. She said her daughter was on a softball team and Margie's mom would always want to watch her granddaughter play ball. One day while walking from the parking lot to the seating area, her mom lost her balance and fell. A trip to the ER and a few sutures later, Margie's mom didn't even remember the episode. Two nights later, there was another game. Margie said that she and her husband were now tightly holding onto her mom's arms while they began to walk. Her mom said to leave her alone;

she is perfectly capable of walking by herself. (Sound familiar?) Margie already knew what could happen if she let go of her mom's arm. Of course, Margie tried to reason with her mom and remind her what happened two nights prior. Her mom didn't remember the incident, doesn't know why she has a bandage on her forehead, and is getting angrier. This was when Margie changed her approach. Rather than telling her mom "what to do," she asked if her mom would help her. Margie stopped, looked at her mom and said, "Mom, let's allow the other parents here to see how proud we are of our little ball player by all locking arms and walking up to the field." Mom looked at Margie and said, "That sounds like fun!"

Your loved-one will often read your body language. This is your expressions, your hands and arms, your voice tone, and even what you are wearing. Most of what a person takes from a conversation comes from your body language. Think about an infant, they take kindly to soothing sounds, gentle stroking, hands and arms reaching out toward them, smiles, songs, and colors like red, green and blue; but not bright yellow. (Physics tells us that more light is reflected by bright colors, resulting in excessive stimulation of the eyes. Hence, painting your walls bright yellow does not often lend to a calming environment.) In approaching our loved-one, keeping a calm voice is the first and most important factor in keeping them at peace. As time progresses, they may no longer remember who you are, so when approaching, you need to understand that they may be afraid. Think about yourself sitting in a seat at the airport while waiting to board your plane and someone walks up to you, calls you Dad, and takes out a napkin and begins to wipe off the corner of your mouth. Or, you are standing when someone walks up and begins to tuck your blouse or shirt into your pants. I don't know about you, but I would find that pretty odd. Imagine the dementia patient that may not know you when you approach them. This is why it is imperative to make sure you are greeted on friendly terms. Start by saying, "Good morning, Mom. You are looking so beautiful this morning. I am here to take you to see Dr. Jones. Can I help you with anything?" Talk in a comforting voice, with a slight smile, and upward turned open outreaching hands. Gentle touching on the arm and back will also help them feel comfortable. This is also a mechanism that subliminally can cause them to move forward. The goal is to get them to do what you need of them, while not causing them to be

To minimize confusion:

1. **Remain calm**
2. **Monitor comfort**
3. **Avoid surprises**

uncomfortable. Wearing colors like blue and green will also cause a calming and restful nature for your loved-one.

Body language in society tells so much about people. Anything from a handshake to arm or leg crossing indicates how welcoming a person is to another. How we stand or sit, physically how close we get within another's personal space, and simple subtle eyebrow lifts all determine a person's interest and comfort with the other. Successful sales people know how to "read the crowd." They can quickly tell if their message is getting received or find their way out.

When your loved-one is trying to communicate with you, be sure to use eye contact, smile, nod your head, respond calmly, and do not point, clench your hands, or fold your arms. It is better to talk slower than to talk louder. Unless a severe hearing condition exists, talking loudly can be construed as scolding or demanding. As the brains degeneration process continues, it can take a little extra time to translate your words into something they can interpret. By using a slower, calming tone, you will have a better chance of being understood by your loved-one. When speaking, be specific; avoid using idioms. "It is raining cats and dogs" can be a bit frightening if taken literally. Unless his reply is, "I know, I stepped in a poodle." Slow and calm at that point may not be needed. I know what I am asking is very hard to do at times, but please believe me that you will nearly always have a better outcome when you follow these engagement steps.

The <u>nurturer</u> is similar to your best friend. The one that always wants the best for you. If you are hungry, they will always feed you. If you need money, they will be there to help. As a nurturing caregiver, you will find that you are putting your loved-one's needs in front of yours, such as the mother feeding the baby before herself. This trait has to be managed carefully. It is quite possible that you will find yourself giving more than you can physically and mentally handle. As you progress through this book, you will learn some ways to help manage this balance.

No matter how strong you might think you are, there is one specific psychological emotional experience that you will deal with for the next several years and that is GUILT. Not sure who invented that stuff, but I am not a fan! Along with guilt is her sister, Shame. Shame is that emotion that might make us happy at first knowing we are doing the right thing but find out from others that we are not.

Making a life-changing decision for a loved-one can create a tremendous amount of guilt; especially, if the action you are requiring of someone is something you know, or at least believe, the other person does not want to have occur. This feeling can become so overwhelming to the point to where you become ill, depressed, cannot sleep, lose your appetite, or get overly angry. We may even become very angry with our loved-one to where we lash out at them or other family members or friends. Guilt very closely mimics the emotions or feeling we have associated with sadness.

We will go through a perfectly logical thought process as to why we have to

> *Guilt and shame are emotions that are overcome by love and forgiveness.*

place our loved-one in a long-term care facility, but the actual action of doing so is where the guilt begins. I can remember for most of my earlier years while living at home, my mother would say that she never wanted to lose her memory and for certain, never wanted to end up in a nursing home. Unfortunately, she would have had better luck buying lottery tickets. Recognizing her wishes, only made it so much more difficult for me to make those tough decisions and the guilt only made it worse. When leaving her long-term care facility from a visit, I would sit in my car in the parking lot and sob out of control. Sometimes I would sit there for 20 - 30 minutes crying over how unfair it is for her to now be trapped in a lifestyle that is completely the opposite of her life-long wishes. Why? Why her? I could always logically justify the move there, however, I couldn't logically justify the pain from the guilt.

Somehow, we feel responsible that our loved-one has dementia, like it is our fault, and now we have been forced to provide the needed care. We convince ourselves that we are causing the worst of a bad situation.

Let's consider the following:

- If the roles were reversed, what would your mom do in providing care for you?
- Are you able to provide better care for your husband than the care facility is providing? Including lifting, bathing, and activities?
- Do you truly feel that you did something wrong, or are you a victim of circumstances?
- Who would you prefer to have oversee your father's care, which sibling or other family member?

- Have you violated your moral code so horribly that you would prefer your loved-one to suffer or have to deal with a degraded quality of life?
- What more could you have done for your mom that she would have approved of if she were able to rationally tell you?
- Are you truly conflicted with guilt knowing you have made the best decisions you could have made in dealing with what you are faced or is the feeling a sense of sadness and sorrow?

It is normal to feel guilt when you know you did something wrong. The way we heal is by accepting our error, make correction, and accept forgiveness.

Then there comes the aunt or sibling who disagrees with your decisions and tries to shame you further into guilt. Lindsey, an amazing woman and a member of my support group, moved across country to live with her mom in order to help with her mother's daily dementia care. After a few months, it became apparent that Lindsey was simply not capable of providing all the care that her mother needed. Her mother was combative, would refuse care, and used language that would have embarrassed Satan. Lindsey called her other siblings and suggested they all consider a long-term care facility for mom. Lindsey's older sister was completely against the idea and began belittling and shaming her. Her sister's comments were, "I cannot understand why you can't do a better job. Mom is not like those actions you have described. It must be something you are doing wrong!" When Lindsey shared these comments with our group, I suggested she instruct her older sister to have mom come move in with her. She followed my advice. The older sister thought that was a terrible idea and cited about five excuses as to why. I then suggested Lindsey tell her sister that she is moving away from mom and back to her home across country; that Lindsey will transfer the power of attorney for healthcare over to the sister; and then use the same excuses as to why she can no longer take care of mom as those her older sister shared for her reasons. Lindsey called her sister and shared this message. Her sister, I guess, had an awakening moment, a shift in her thinking (my dad would call this "a trip to the woodshed") and began back peddling. Once Lindsey' sister realized that her mother was going to be left on her own and if even half of what Lindsey reported was true, this older sister would be receiving phone calls continuously. Amazingly, her sister became complimentary and grateful for what Lindsey was doing and said she would support the decision if a move to a long-term care facility was what was needed for Mom. Lindsey placed her mom in a long-term care facility and all family members were at peace. About a month later, her older sister came to town to visit the mother and was actually able to observe much of what Lindsey had reported. Her sister's response, "I had no idea what you were going through! Mom didn't even remember my name." she said crying.

A quick side note; there are reasons and there are excuses. Reasons are based on factual information. "I could not attend your party because I was in the hospital." Excuses are based on decisions. Excuses are

> *Reasons are factual and truthful. Excuses mean a person does not want to help you..*

lies, deceit, laziness, lack of interest, … "I could not attend your party because I had to clean my house." Fact is, if you wanted to attend the party, you could clean the house at a different time. When you are told by your brother that he cannot help care for mom during your surgery citing that he will be camping in the mountains, remember, if taking care of mom were of utmost importance to him, he could reschedule his camping trip to a different time.

You will be making many decisions that will not please everyone. You will be making decisions that will not please your loved-one. These decisions need to be made. Hopefully with the guidance of this book, you will be better armed to make the best decision possible. The guilt and shame will weigh on you. Please recognize and accept why you have to make these decisions, popular or not. George Foreman once said, "I was a tiger, a good fighter, in good shape, but I was always nervous before boxing matches."

I am hoping you understand that in placing your loved-one into a care facility, you are not at fault. This is simply an unfortunate, necessary step in providing quality care. Remember, **caregiving is not an obligation; it is a privilege**. I look back at the time I spent with my mom and remember how much of an honor it was and something I will never forget, that I was the one holding her hand when she took her final breath.

Fear and Ought

While you are trying to manage your way through the guilt and shame cycle, you will likely also face the fear of failure and the "Ought Syndrome." Benjamin Franklin said there are only two things certain in life: death and taxes. I would add a third certainty; change. Change is the component that you as a caregiver will have to allow. Your loved-one is undergoing massive change, so you will have to adapt. This is where the fear of failure comes in. Let me assure you that you will fail at times. As with most challenges, we must simply

> *Caring for a person with dementia is not about perfection, it is about love.*

keep trying. We may say or do something, then soon realize it was wrong. So, let's just agree to not do that again and move on. Caring for a person with dementia is not about perfection, it is about love. As we continue to love, we will continue to try to be the best we can be. It is entirely possible that they will not remember the mistake and you are good to move on.

There is the "fear of failure" and there is the "fear of what is to come." The fear of what is to come will completely wear you down if you let it. I promise that if that day or event that you have been fearing comes to fruition, it will be nothing at all like you expected or worried about over the past days, months, years. Right now, you can only control what is in your power to control. Fear is an emotion that disrupts logical thinking. By allowing fear to control you, it will cause you to make mistakes. I believe you will have a greater level of preparedness and make fewer mistakes by reading through this book. So please fear not.

Once you accept the fact that you will fail from time to time and no one went to jail or landed in the hospital as a result of the fail, then move on. If you don't you will find yourself dealing with the Ought Syndrome. This is my term for the "What I ought to have done," or "I ought to do ...", conditions. You begin to second guess yourself on everything. Whatever it is that you think should be one way, you will think of two or three other ways of doing it until you do nothing and realize that you ought to have at least done something. There are those times where you will even say, "I should ought to have not done that." This book should help clarify your ought's, not's, and fear's.

And finally, how often do we think that we will get to it tomorrow. And when we wake up the next morning, suddenly it is today. Somehow, tomorrow didn't occur. If we spend time preparing, in place of worry, fear, or ought's, we can then expect a more successful outcome. A lack of preparation on your part <u>will</u> constitute an emergency on the part of someone else. The intent of this book is to step you along that path. I am hopeful it will navigate you through the multitude of challenges and changes you will experience in caring and loving the one that is entrusting their life to you.

And Now for Some Ground-Rules to Follow...

I would provide all new members to the support group the following list of rules or guidelines that we as a group would enlist as our discussion baseline. This list is a quick primer to help the new members get started with their journey while starting conversations.

1. **Inform loved-one of diagnosis.** Everyone is entitled to know what is medically wrong with them. In fact, I believe a medical professional has an obligation to be upfront and honest with their patients. Regardless of whether we simply have the common cold or Alzheimer's, the doctor has an obligation to tell us the diagnosis. At that time, we have the choice to follow their prescribed care routine or to ignore it as if it will eventually go away. I believe a dementia victim must be told of his prognosis, offered the proper diagnostic testing to properly evaluate the symptoms (or at least eliminate some of the things that it is not), and prescribed care that will either heal or at least comfort the patient.

When dealing with dementia, you can choose to keep reminding the patient that they cannot remember or take a different path. People have difficulty in accepting they have a mental disorder. In fact, it is probably the most common remark that you can tell someone that will get the greatest denial. Even though the doctor says they have dementia and we remind them they have dementia, they will reply with a "there is nothing wrong with my memory." They have been told, so let's leave it at that. Continual reminding only threatens your relationship. Forget "remember".

2. They lose the ability to do rational thinking. They eventually lose the ability to process methods or learn new procedures. Rational thinking is where an individual will think in a logically consistent way.

Rational thinking does not exist in an irrational mind.

Methods and procedures usually follow a logical sequence. Some methods and procedures can become a muscle memory; we can do these things without thought. New methods and procedures require a memorization of a pattern of steps. There comes a point where no matter how hard you try or how angry you get, you will not be able to teach your loved-one how to use that remote control for the new, much larger television you just bought them thinking you were helping them better see the evening news.

My mom was the best cook in the world. (I know this is disappointing for many of you to hear thinking you maintain that title.) When visiting her one evening, I commented to her, "I smell paint." and asked her if someone in her building was doing some painting. She was not sure. A little while later, my wife, our two children, my mom, and I sat down for dinner. After completing the main course, she got up and said she made some pumpkin pie for dessert. This was quite pleasing to my ears, and belly. After setting a piece of pie in front of us, we all took a bite. My family immediately looked at each other, my son and daughter let their bites in their mouths fall out onto their plates, my wife and I swallowed our bite. I discovered the source of the paint smell. The three of them commented that they are very full. I, not wanting to disappoint my mom, finished my entire piece. Soon after dishes were done and all retired to the living room, I went on a mission. The first thing I did was open the can of vegetable shortening. BINGO! Once I was able to regain control of my vision from taking a big smell of the can's contents, I quickly recapped the can. Apparently cooking products have a shelf-life. A can of vegetable shortening that expired 5-years prior, I came to learn, is best not to be used for cooking a pie. Let alone anything! I slipped off to the grocery store, purchased a "fresh" can of vegetable shortening, and threw away the rancid one.

My mom was capable of making a pie just as she had for 60+ years. Her dementia caused her to overlook one minor detail. This detail was one that had she been more capable of evaluating the process, could have been avoided.

3. Maintain optimism. If I were to tell you that you have a terminal illness and that you have a few months or even a few years to live, how would this make you feel? In a rational world, you may become severely depressed, eventually begin to get your affairs in order, and make a plan to do or see things you've wanted to see or accomplish before death. Those living in the "normal" world have the ability to vacation to tropical locations, watch children graduate with honors, see and hold that beautiful new granddaughter, sit on the back porch and watch the setting sun as it radiates the sky with a spectrum of color, have a candlelit dinner with your special sweetie, and receive that special hug and kiss from the person with whom you have chosen to spend your years. Now when you live in a non-rational thinking world, you have a limited capacity in making plans or achieving goals. You are no longer in control of your destiny; someone else must either help with the planning and attaining of these objectives or they will not occur. People react in a positive fashion if they have something to look forward to.

Continual reminders of, "You have Alzheimer's, that is why you are going to the nursing home," certainly does not build character. I believe we need to be positive and optimistic in dealing with dementia victims. If it means redirecting or readjusting the message, we must never give the patient the feeling they have a memory condition that will eventually take their life. They have already been told this. There is no need to keep reminding them.

When my mom was in her long-term care facility, she kept asking me when she would be able to go home. What do you think her reaction would be if I told her that she was going to be at this facility until it takes her life? Likely that would be the case but telling her that and reinforcing that would be horrific for her. In order to try to be more uplifting, I said that the doctor wants her at this facility until she can begin walking on her own again. Her comment, "Why there is nothing wrong with my walking, I can walk through that window right now." With a slight smirk, I thought, and that is why you are here. The point is, I gave her hope.

4. Support a good quality of life. Everyone is entitled to quality of life. Just because these people may have become a "shell," which is a term that is commonly used; they still have a mind, a soul, and a heart. Although we have difficulty communicating with them and, at times it drives us nuts, it is no reason to think anything less of them. There is a program called Namaste, developed by Joyce Simard, which provides for social interactions with patients in their late term. Namaste is a Hindu term meaning,

Maintaining Quality of Life, Dignity, and Optimism are critical in trying to provide your loved-one with a manageable mental state.

"to honor the spirit within." Many of these folks she works with are those that we often see just sitting in a wheelchair, slumped over, sleeping, and often drooling upon themselves. Sometimes, these folks have not seen loved-ones for months and have not smiled for years. We are challenged, because we do not know what to do with or around these folks. Namaste engages with these people by touching their soul. It is a technique that includes touching, hugging, aromatherapy, lotions, and eye contact. Some nursing homes have begun adopting these principles and have experienced amazing results. The net outcome is an improved quality of life. Are these folks not allowed to have dignity? Should we just put them in a corner and ignore them while waiting for them to die?

Richard, a regular attendee of the support group, said his mother loves hugs. He said that she will have a complete change in demeaner following a good hug. Several university studies have determined a measurable therapeutic value associated with good and frequent hugs. These hugs can reduce stress, lower blood pressure, improve immune function and strengthen pain tolerance. Lisa told us that she has developed a technique that she calls the 20-Second Hug. It starts with holding each other together tightly and then start counting; 1-I love you, 2-I love you, 3-I love you... She said that when doing this with her husband and they get to 20 she will say something like "until the end of time," or "forever and ever."

Lisa added that her husband has not been speaking much, but one day when they got to 20, he said, "as long as the stars continue to twinkle in the sky." She fell to her knees in tears of joy.

5. Validate, validate, validate. I prefer the term "Therapeutic Fibbing." I always get criticized on this one. New members will tell me that they cannot and will not lie to their loved-one. One week I actually got into a biblical discussion with a retired Baptist pastor explaining to him that I am not suggesting he lie to his wife. I suggested he may consider defining the term lie to be if you intentionally mean to deceive another party to protect your reputation or to try to cover up or hide the truth for personal gain. He wasn't buying it. I said in the case of "Therapeutic Fibbing," we are sometimes avoiding the truth or only telling part of the truth. Overall, this process supports quality of life standards and provides for optimism. You can say that I have never lied to my wife and I am not going to start now. Good luck with that. I assure you by taking this approach, no one wins. In fact, you will find you are not helping in

If you take away only one thing from this book, I urge you to master "Therapeutic Fibbing."

maintaining their quality of life, that very thing they are counting on you to help provide.

I ask you to not judge me here. I actually am a very honest guy. I am suggesting that when your wife asks, "Why do I have to take all these pills?" to not tell her that the little round one is for her memory. And, in particular, if she is in denial of having memory problems. Stick with me on this for a bit longer, I believe you see why this tool is very valuable and provides for that quality of life. By the way, the Baptist pastor is now an endorser of this technique.

6. Cleanliness is not Godliness. Pick your battles. Is it truly all that important that they have bathed or shaved today? You are not going anywhere, no one is coming over, it is just you and your loved-one at home. Certainly, staying sanitary is always important; but sometimes dealing with the trauma associated with the bath or shower may not be something you need to deal with more than one or two times a week.

I would hear this issue mentioned monthly from one of our group members regarding their loved-one.

7. Forget "remember." (Have you heard this expression somewhere before?) Remove the term "remember" from your conversations. We say, "Remember when..." or "Why can't you remember the...." This is only a reminder that they are having difficulty. It would be like having a family member restricted to a wheelchair and then asking them to go skiing or maybe mountain climbing. These are simply bad reminders. Work on removing the term "remember" from your vocabulary. Trust me; less stress for both of you.

A second word to remove from your daily use is "Why." When we ask a question beginning with "Why," are we actually expecting an answer? "Why did you put your shirt on inside-out?" "Why didn't you eat the lunch I prepared for you?" We already know the answer before we ask it so let's try to avoid creating more confusion while reminding them once again that they have a memory issue.

Forget "remember" and "why". (I am hoping you did not just pick up the book and begin reading with that sentence.)

 8. **It is okay for YOU to forget.** When your loved-one suddenly has a surge of clarity and remembers something you promised, thinking they would not remember; it is OK for you to say, "I forgot." It carries more meaning if you act sincere, not so much though if you are telling the tax-collector you forgot to pay your taxes. Your loved-one may be a bit upset

when you forget something but will forgive and all is well.

9. Take care of yourself. You are part of a very important triad, your loved-one, the doctor, and you. We often think that their care is our key focus. When actually the most important link is you. Without you, everything falls apart. If we fail to check the oil in our car, if we see the temperature gauge rising on the dash panel, or if we pass up that gas station saying that we can probably make it to the next station before we actually have to stop; all lead to disaster. Likewise, we must keep ourselves in top running order. If OUR health is weakened, so is the care we can provide.

10. The doctor is not the boss. It is always easy to blame the doctor for your health care issues, but underneath it all, the final decision is yours. It is up

Alzheimer's will not wait for you!

to you to decide if you are going to follow the doctor's directives. Are we going to follow them to the letter or are we going to do what he said for a day or two and then say, OK I feel fine now, and stop? You have to take responsibility for your own care. You also are responsible for the care of your loved-one. The doctor is not in charge of your life or the life of your loved-one. And, sometimes we have to fire a doctor. Sometimes the doctor is wrong. It is advisable, if you are going to deviate from the doctor's orders, that you seek alternative professional medical advice. Never ignore or brush-off a medical diagnosis. Your doctor's opinion is based on something. If you are not happy, go to another doctor or medical specialist.

Notes:

SECTION 2

This section is designed to help you accomplish many of the necessary issues you will need to deal with over the next several months to years. I have always been a believer in that **if you wake up without a plan, someone will make one for you.** It is better to have a plan and not need it than not to have a plan and urgently need one. This material is a creation of multiple years of listening, study, and research. I identify this section as my 13 Steps to Care. As a caregiver, a family member, advisor, medical professional, friend, or the one with dementia; these steps are critical in getting you and your loved-one from today to where your involvement becomes minimized. If you specifically are not the one that will take on one or all of the 13 Steps listed, I assure you, it will still need done by someone. Please remember, you will have your own unique set of circumstances that may not follow these exact guidelines I have prescribed. You may need to look at these specific steps as recommendations or suggestions and then make any needed adjustments based on your specific circumstances. No two Alzheimer's patients are identical. No two caregivers are identical.

13 Steps to Care

I was asked by a group member if there was a step-by-step list of activities that would help her know what is next. She said that she needs to plan and be prepared for what is to come. From her request, I formed the following, 13 Steps to Care, to use as discussion topics within our group. As I began to write this book, it occurred to me that if a caregiver can become familiar with these very important and invaluable steps, the future direction will be clearer and better defined. Everyone who is helping another person in managing their pathway through the various traumatic dementia challenges will be faced with each of these 13 Steps. I have taken each of these 13 Steps and am providing you with enrichment and thought so as to help improve YOUR quality of life. By following these 13 Steps to Care, you will not be alone. You will have at least a suggestion to help you get started.

1. Get Diagnosis – Definitive

The very first step to care is to understand what you are dealing with. All too often, we think of memory problems as a normal part of aging. For years, it was senility, insanity, hardening of the arteries, softening of the brain, and mania. Thanks to modern science, research has been able to better identify and define the various forms of dementia. Some dementias may be hereditary. Alzheimer's disease has not been conclusively proven to be hereditary. According to the National Institute on Aging, we learn there is a gene relationship associated with Early-onset Alzheimer's. It is reported that it is caused by mutations on chromosomes 21, 14, and 1. Each mutation causes abnormal proteins to develop. The proteins are a part of the development of the amyloid plaques, present in the brain of an Alzheimer's patient. Research says that less than 10% of people with Alzheimer's are affected with the Early-onset. This can affect a person in his 30's to mid-60's and can be considered inherited. On the other hand,

When Cognitive impairment can may be mistaken for dementia:

- **UTI**
- **Depression**
- **Normal Pressure Hydrocephalus**
- **Subdural Hematoma**

having these genetic markers does not mean that you will be inflicted with Alzheimer's. Individuals displaying symptoms in their mid-60's and later, fall into Late-onset Alzheimer's. Another genetic marker, a protein APOE ε4 on chromosome 19 seems to put a person at greater risk than one with the APOE ε2 or the APOE ε3 protein. Again, everyone is different and can react differently to these proteins.

Alzheimer's disease affects memory first and later progresses to affect the brain's other cognitive skills, such as speech, ability to reason, movement, and motor skills. Interestingly, very old "procedural memories", such as playing the piano, may be retained beyond the patient's ability to recognize their closest family member.

Vascular dementia, formerly known as Multi-Infarct Dementia results following a minor stroke(s) in the brain causing irreversible damage. A precursor to the stroke may be the Transient Ischemic Attack (TIA). The TIA can be a warning sign of an upcoming stroke. The symptoms will depend upon which area of the brain is affected; often it is the memory and other cognitive functions, similar to that of Alzheimer's with the exception of the late-term characteristics of Alzheimer's. The Alzheimer's Association tells us that our brain is nourished by one of our body's richest networks of blood vessels. Anything that damages blood vessels anywhere in our body can damage blood vessels in our brain, depriving brain cells of vital food and oxygen. Blood vessel changes in the brain are linked to vascular dementia. They often are present along with changes caused by other types of dementia, including Alzheimer's disease and dementia with Lewy bodies. These changes may interact to cause faster decline or make impairments more severe. We can help protect our brain with some of the same strategies that protect our heart — don't smoke; take steps to keep our blood pressure, cholesterol and blood sugar within recommended limits; maintain a healthy weight; and exercise three to four times a week. (Sorry, for mentioning the "e-word.")

Dementia with Lewy bodies DLB, now the third most common cause of dementia and the most misdiagnosed, presents itself as a decrease in cognitive ability, hallucinations, movement problems, and delusions. Parkinson's symptoms, such as hunched posture, rigid muscles and balance are also seen as characteristics of Lewy bodies. Frontotemporal Dementias, FTD, (once known as Pick's disease but redefined as a subtype) affects personality (inhibitions), inappropriate or indifferent behavior, and speech, like finding the right word, but not memory. Frontotemporal dementia usually appears between the ages of 45 and 65, while Alzheimer's more often appears after age 65.

A key fact to remember, **it is very possible to have more than one dementia type.** For example, your loved-one can have both Vascular dementia and Alzheimer's simultaneously.

> *It is very possible to have more than one dementia type.*

As a child or sibling of someone with a dementia, wouldn't it be nice to know what you may have in store for your future? Would it be possible to prevent or minimize the likelihood of you contracting the same disease? What would it be worth to you to know what you need to add or avoid to potentially stay-off a dementia condition? More than likely, steps can be taken earlier in life that may help avoid the onset of the disease. Although, we still do not have a one hundred percent conclusive mechanism to test for Alzheimer's, the medical community often just assumes the patient has Alzheimer's along with any other already-determined dementia. After thorough testing and all other dementias have been eliminated, doctors conclude that it is Alzheimer's. Some doctors will assume it is Alzheimer's without further testing. There are drugs prescribed specifically for Alzheimer's and nothing else. Due to the indecisiveness of the disease, some doctors will prescribe these drugs as part of the overall regime of medications. These drugs are often administered earlier than recommended by the drug companies.

Vascular dementia patients often have a common thread and that is elevated levels of cholesterol within their blood. A recent study concluded that even moderately elevated cholesterol increased dementia risk.

Frequently, when I ask people if they have gotten a diagnosis for their loved-one, the reply is, "His doctor gave him the Mini-Mental State Exam (MMSE) and believes it to be dementia possibly Alzheimer's." (The MMSE is a widely-used tool for tracking dementia.) Then the doctor gave them some Aricept (Donepezil) and sent them on their way. The frustrating issue at hand is that this cognitive test can be very subjective and should not be the only tool used in detecting earlier-stage memory loss. There are so many other factors that can create a dementia-like effect that a skills test can lend itself inadequate at times. Simple fear of tests can be enough to cause someone to score poorly. Dehydration or severe anxiety can cause a dementia-like state. Not to mention that the person may just be illiterate or have a low IQ. I had a lady come up to me after one of my speaking engagements, Mary suggest that she believes her husband may have Alzheimer's. I asked Mary if a diagnosis had been provided by a physician. She said that the doctor told her that if her husband was capable of driving home, then there is nothing wrong with him. Of course, I asked her if she asked the doctor to ride home with him or better yet, walk out in front of the car while he is approaching. She responded that she will next time. So now this poor woman has to deal with her husband resting on the laurels of the doctor's possible misleading findings. Meanwhile, Mary has to continue listening to him tell the same story over and over. She has to argue with him about meals and bathing. Mary has the constant fear that he may forget where to find the brake pedal in the car. Not only could he be injured, but he could also harm someone else.

If I had a toothache, would it be wise to go to a podiatrist? The human body is a very complex organism. To complicate it further, our body's chemistry continues to change as we age. The body comes in different ethnic varieties and genders.

General Practitioners, the "family doctor", are very good at knowing a little bit about a lot. However, it is impractical to think your family doctor is as effective in dealing with an infant as he would be with a 90-year old woman. The GP is trained to identify conditions and diagnose treatment. Can most spot dementia symptoms? Of course, they can. Are they capable of properly treating a dementia patient? Considering the multitude of dementias, I would suggest this is not their specialty. Your GP's role is to prescribe closer evaluation from someone skilled in that area of medicine; such as a neurologist. In Mary's case, her husband was only 54-years old. The doctor could have suggested he have an MRI (Magnetic Resonance Imaging) and possibly visit a psychiatrist. It is fairly uncommon for a man his age to be experiencing a degenerative dementia. Depression and psychosis are also conditions that can allow for dementia-like symptoms. Even vitamin deficiencies and infections commonly cause confusion or disorientation in the elderly. A visit with a psychiatrist can help identify several types of neurotic disorders, if present. Once properly diagnosed as a non-curable dementia, is a psychiatrist then the best option? I would encourage you discuss this in depth with your primary care physician or your neurologist.

Some people are blessed with a loved-one that is willing to go to a doctor for evaluation and seek a diagnosis. If this is the case with the one you are caring for, you are very fortunate. Often though, I have people tell me that their loved-one refuses to go to the doctor and there is nothing they can do about it. They say that the person will fight them if necessary. This is a perfect example as to why I recommend getting them evaluated as soon as the first symptoms are noticed. As time progresses, their ability to do rational thinking diminishes; combine this with some psychotic behavioral changes and you may find it easier to walk through a lion's cage with a pork chop hanging around your neck. Let's look at this problem from two directions, first the early-stage-early-detection victim and second the mean, ornery patient that will require most of the Army's 5th Infantry to get him out of the house. For our first example, the loved-one will be more understanding and supportive of going to a doctor if their trusted advisor asks or tells them to do so. Otherwise, a little persuasion may be necessary. This can be done by offering a simple bribe, something like, "If you go to the doctor, we will get some ice cream on the way home." Or maybe go to the park, mall, Home Depot, whatever you think might incentivize them.

Your GP may not be the "right" doctor, but certainly should be the first stop. Ask your GP for a recommendation for a geriatrician if the GP feels his skills do not lend well to dementia care. The geriatrician is trained to work with elderly patients. If the GP recognizes some dementia, a recommendation for a neurologist is also a wonderful idea. Sometimes the GP does not want to give up the business, if this becomes your experience, you can contact your local Alzheimer's Association for recommendations or ask friends for references. I mentioned earlier in this section the Mini-Mental State Exam (MMSE) used for cognitive assessments; this would be only one step in assuming the diagnosis. Insist on further testing, these can include MRI (magnetic resonance imaging), CT scan (computed tomography), and PET scan (positron emission tomography).

There can be up to a 20% discrepancy between the clinical diagnosis of Alzheimer's disease and the pathological diagnosis.

Remember, Alzheimer's can only be diagnosed by a process of elimination. Your loved-one's health is far too important. Another reason why you want to get a thorough evaluation done as soon as possible is that the longer we can prolong a stable condition for your loved-one, the better the chances are that more effective medicine will become available, and hopefully a cure.

Now let's look at the patient that would rather fight than seek medical attention. There comes a time where we have to become more forceful, not in a violent manner, but to show the person we will not take "no" for an answer. We may need to resort to threats, a stern voice, strong eye contact, or even punishment (nothing physical). You will try to reason with the person, but if you recall and I know you do, trying to be rational with your loved-one is futile. You may need to tell them, "Either get to the doctor or pack your bags and get out." I have never heard of anyone actually contacting a moving company to come help them move. You can sit them down, look into their eyes, with your finger pointed, tell them, "I love you very much. By you choosing not going to the doctor, hurts me. I am telling you to go." And if you really want to make a big splash, "Either you go to the doctor on your own, or I will have the police take you." I find that when the patient sees that they are out-gunned, they tend to back down. In extreme cases, you may have to solicit the help of the police. I am friends with Martha. She was caring for her husband, retired military. Martha would tell her husband if he did not follow up with proper medical attention that she would report him to his commanding officer. Of course, his commanding officer, if still around, would not be of much help, but Martha's husband could not rationally figure that out. Another fallback that I have seen work, "If you go with me to visit your doctor, we will stop and get ice cream on the way home." Personally, I think I would do just about anything for a bowl of ice cream.

It helps to take your loved-one to a doctor they trust. Then, this doctor can become the "bad guy." This "trusted doctor" can then tell the patient to take medicine, stop driving, or seek additional care. You need to get a copy of all the doctor's orders. This then can be used later when your loved-one questions why they have to do something. You pull out the note and blame it on the doctor. As I mentioned, by blaming it on the doctor, it keeps you from having to be the disciplinarian. In ultimately extreme cases, you can get a court order demanding he visits a primary care physician. I have never heard of anyone having to resort to this extreme, and I would assume it would also include you obtaining guardianship. Eek! I'll talk about this later.

So, we have managed to get the loved-one to a doctor and or a referral to a geriatrician. You will probably have to sit through the MMSE, your loved-one will probably fail. As I said, I would probably fail the test as well. Although I can count backwards by 7/4's, I cannot seem to remember someone's name by the time I get done shaking his hand. Regardless, the doctor will probably start the patient on something like Aricept (Donepezil), Razadyne (Galantamine), or Exelon (Rivastigmine); cholinesterase inhibitors. Often enough, the doctor also starts Namenda (Memantine) at the same time. We will discuss this drug later. Another medication, Namzaric, combines the cholinesterase inhibitor with the memantine. The doctor may then ask you to come back in three months. Here is where I suggest you tell the doctor that you want a diagnosis. The doctor will probably say something like dementia blah, blah, blah. Now is where you can show the doctor that you have done your homework. You respectfully say to the doctor, "You know Doc, there are nearly one hundred different types of dementia. I am not sure you have been able to quite narrow the playing field by just asking my loved-one a few questions. Wouldn't you think a blood test would be in order, should we do a Vitamin B12 screening, and why haven't you suggested a neurologist or a geriatrician?" You will find the doctor quickly writing scripts for further testing. If the doctor says there is no need for any of these additional tests, then I would like his name because I will have him buy me some lottery tickets since he apparently has psychic powers. Otherwise, I would wonder why the doctor believes your loved-one is not deserving of further testing and ultimately a diagnosis. I tend to believe that if the doctor's mother had "just dementia" that he would be a little more responsive. Note: Always be mindful of the doctor to patient relationship in making your decisions. Burning bridges are not often your best option.

Clinical diagnosis is based upon signs, symptoms, and medical history. A pathological diagnosis is based upon lab tests and medical imaging.

You now have an order to get some further testing or at least a referral to a physician that can more closely evaluate the form and severity of the dementia. Hopefully you did not have to leave the doctor looking like Beetle Bailey after the Sarge finished with him. Remember, we are not talking about repairs to your car, this is your loved-one; in many cases, the most important person in your life.

Your local Alzheimer's Association can refer some neurologists and geriatricians in your area that work well with elderly folks. Be prepared; when you call the neurologist, they will probably tell you there is a one to two month wait before your first visit. I am quite concerned that as more and more Baby Boomers start entering into their late 70's and 80's that there will be nowhere near enough neurologists to go around.

Your neurologist or geriatrician will probably start with another round of the MMSE test; lucky for you. However, they will normally then order more extensive testing best suited to the characteristics of your loved-one. As I keep stating, Alzheimer's is determined by a process of elimination. It is important to weed through all the other dementia's before finalizing on Alzheimer's. From this point forward, the physician will be the person you will go to for all brain health issues and including any type of psychotic display your loved-one may present.

If you happen to be working with a geriatrician, they may likely do all the proper testing, both blood and non-invasive imaging, in order to best determine what they are dealing with. In my investigations, I found that the geriatrician will not prescribe the neurologist's services if the testing concludes actual age-related dementia. If a condition is determined curable, a neurologist will likely be the proper choice and referred by the geriatrician.

2. Acceptance

The one, and most important, step in the entire process is the complete acceptance of the problem. Care cannot begin until you, as a caregiver, have accepted the problem. This is true in dealing with any type of disease. As long as you choose to deny or ignore the symptoms the longer it will be before your loved-one can get care. The amount of time spent in denial can be horrendous. Although it is very helpful when the victim recognizes

> *Complete acceptance is an action phrase meaning a non-conditional conscious commitment to a process or condition.*

changes and is willing and wanting to learn about what is happening and looking for help. It is very important for you as a loved-one, the trusted advisor, to get on board immediately. As the expression goes, **"you have to be all in!"** You can play it down, you can avoid and or ignore that something is wrong, but guess what? The problem will not go away...in fact it gets worse. Don't fall into the Ought Syndrome. Not to mention if the problem is related to something that is curable, think of how you will feel having put yourself and your loved-one through the torment. This can be compared to a heart attack. How often do people ignore the symptoms? How many people could have avoided the trauma, not to mention death, if they had only listened to their bodies? The early warning signs listed earlier are important indicators of our body telling us there is something wrong. If your loved-one is only experiencing one of the 10 Warning Signs of Alzheimer's as identified in Section 1, it is possible that some other environmental, chemical, or physiological condition may exist. Allergies, diet, stress, and lack of sleep are common reasons for forgetfulness or mood changes. Medicines, poor blood flow, and reduced oxygen intake effect judgment and initiative. However, if your loved-one displays three and four of these symptoms, I definitely think professional attention would be in order.

When the loved-one has many family members, often this introduces complexity. For example, let's look at the "Nelson" family. Dad is demonstrating signs of dementia. Mom is the primary caregiver while one of the daughters, Sara, helps Mom with activities like taking Dad to the doctor and does the grocery shopping. Another daughter has her own family and is "just too busy" to help. One son lives out-of-state and the other lives just across town. Dad's sister is already in a Long-Term Care facility. This sounds like an odd circumstance, but please believe me when

I say that I have seen this scenario more times than I care to count. To define the illustration further, the son from out-of-town rarely sees Dad, but talks to him on the phone and agrees that Dad has changed a bit. The son across town is fully in denial. There is nothing wrong with Dad, he is just getting old, he has a lot on his mind, and everyone is picking on him. The "too busy" daughter is also in denial, knows something is changing with Dad, but is too frightened to the point that she feels unable help. The helping daughter, Sara, is there for Mom and Dad and wants to get

Denial is an unconscious state characterized by refusal to accept painful realities.

more help for Dad. Sara is perceived by a few of her siblings to be mainly concerned about the inheritance; she just wants Mom and Dad's money. Maybe some of this is beginning to sound similar to your family. Mom has noticed changes in Dad that extend back a couple years but has not said anything to anyone else. In fact, she has done a great job in helping to mask the symptoms. Have you ever heard two people talking where one of the folks always fills in a word or two? This is a way of masking symptoms. He says, "I need to fix that lamp in the living room. I think I will go to, um." "Home Depot" the woman quickly adds. "Yeah, Home Depot," he replies. Another example,

"Honey, the grandkids just got here. Let's give Justin, Robin, and Rachel big hugs." Any chance he would not have remembered the names without her input? And, "Oh thank you so much for coming to visit. Bill say goodbye to Karen." These fillers all seem innocent and often done subconsciously. You can see, though, why someone not witnessing Dad's behavior 24/7 can come to the conclusion that there is nothing wrong, Dad is fine.

As desirable as it might be to have the whole family working in unison, it is often not the case. Who suffers? Dad? Mom? The siblings? The right answer is everyone. Dad, of course, because Mom is afraid to seek adequate medical attention without the family's blessing. After all, her son across town is a strong character and not afraid to let Mom know how he feels about the whole mess. Mom is getting beaten down because of Dad's continual questions, his wanting to drive, he's making crazy money decisions, and the unsolicited pressure she gets from her wonderful, but difficult son. The siblings are losing their Dad. All of them know something is wrong, they have heard of Alzheimer's, and they know what the long-term effect will mean. **This is the long goodbye.** I am sure by reading this example, it is clear what needs to be done; unless of course this is your family. In that event, I will continue. To explain, let's first agree on who is the most important person in the example I just provided. Dad? Mom? Helpful daughter? Too busy daughter? Out-of-town son? Or in-town, pain in the patootie son? Survey says...if you guessed Dad, you have just lost your chance at the bonus round. If you guessed any of the children; thank you for playing but you will be going home empty-handed. If you guessed the Mom, you are right. You instantly advance to the Winners Circle. Mom is the glue, the conduit connecting Dad to everything else. If Mom is ill or if Mom is not in the picture, the responsibility falls to one of the children for this task. It is important to remember, Mom needs to stay healthy. And, Mom needs some time alone.

Let's take a look at the children and learn how to whip them into shape. (My dad would refer to it as a trip to the woodshed.) Frequently, as people age, their children become a stronger, more vocal part of the union or family. Elderly folks will, at times, yield to their children and follow their direction or suggestion. In the case of the Nelson family, listed here, it is important for one of the children to take the lead. If the Nelson's were to let patootie-son take the lead, the outcome could lead to grave consequences.

Who is the oldest? Which child has assumed the lead in other family functions? This is a way of determining who should be the "voice" of the family. Obviously, the "voice" has to be in agreement that Dad needs immediate attention. As for the Nelson's, they determined that the out-of-town son was actually the one that would assume the lead role. Recognizing he is not local, he may need to come to town for a family meeting or will have to conduct discussions over the phone.

> **Denial and greed are two evils that tear families apart.**

His job will be to TELL others in the family their roles and responsibilities. If one or more of the children decides that they will not play in his sandbox, they will need to be instructed to get out. This whole issue cannot be taken lightly and there is no time for popularity contests. Dad has a problem and Mom needs our support. If helpful-daughter can and will continue the course, that would be fantastic. If too-busy-daughter chooses to keep away, she needs to be informed that her help and support is needed and appreciated, but otherwise do not get in the way. Patootie-son, oh yes, I leave the best for last. We all love him, we know he means well, but in life there is a saying, "You are either part of the problem or part of the solution." This young man needs to decide which role he would like to play.

If he chooses to be part of the problem, he is told if he interferes with Dad's care or continues to intimidate Mom, legal action will occur if necessary. I know you don't want to tell your brother if he doesn't play nice you are going to get him in trouble, but you are talking about your Mom's health and wellbeing. Of course, there is the option where Dad can move in with him and he can then become the primary caregiver. As often as I have heard this threat given to another family member, I have yet to hear of the action actually occurring. You will find patootie-son has dozens of reasons why he cannot make that happen. You will hear excuses such as work, soccer, travel, Dad snores too loud, or being a burden on his family. It is much easier to be critical of Mom than it would be for him to takeover. Give it some time. Dad will regress further, and it will become very obvious how wrong this son was in his assessment in suggesting there was nothing wrong with Dad and therefore should delay treatment.

Too-busy-daughter is often a common trait within a family. A lot of times, it is legitimate. This daughter may work full time, have children active in sports and school activities, and her husband has frequent trips associated with his job. However, the characteristic with this type of person is typically still one that will have the folks over for dinner on Sunday or try to pick up Dad and take him to watch his grandson kick that winning goal. On the flip side, this daughter may be so overwhelmed and scared of what is happening to Dad that she slips into a shell. It is easier to avoid the issue by "creating" excuses than to take a proactive role. Even family get-togethers will often see this daughter not in attendance. It is typical for other family members to get angry with her,

No one is born a caregiver.

arguing that she is not being responsive to Mom and Dad. I know this situation is sad. Sometimes there are lingering feelings as to why she does not want to help. As I mentioned earlier, we are not born caregivers. Just because I am not able either mentally or physically to help my loved-one, does not mean that I love them any less than someone else does. It simply means that I am incapable of helping. Should we just say, "Oh well" and move on? No. There are still things that we can do that can engage this sister/daughter that will help her feel involved while working for a common cause. She can do some simple things like cut coupons for grocery items for the folks. As time progresses, the patient will need products like Boost and Depends. Coupons are often hard to find, but by saving money on other grocery items, helps offset the total costs. This daughter can join a wholesale club where she can help even further by getting many of the common items for a reduced price. You will probably find that the too-busy-daughter's children are eager to help shop for Grandma and Grandpa. Mom may still need to shop for some items like milk, meats, and pharmaceuticals, but for the most part, this daughter will have been a big help. As the loved-one progresses through the disease's process, their interests will change. This daughter can help put together a collection of old movies for Dad. She can assemble a collection of gospel music or hymns for Dad. Videos of past football games, baseball games, and even golf matches are ideas of interest. I have seen some very interested in cartoons like Tom and Jerry, Bugs Bunny, and Road Runner. With today's technology, all of this can be collected and assembled for almost nothing. You can experiment as to Dad's interests and attentiveness by renting a DVD from the library. They have old movies, sports, and cartoons all on DVD. Even old war movies or documentaries could peak his interests. The daughter can take items to the drycleaners, the grandkids can cut the grass, rake leaves, shovel snow, in fact once a week, her family can make a dinner or even bake a cake for Grandma and Grandpa. I think you will find that if you can give this daughter small, manageable tasks, she will come around.

Let's move away from the Nelson family now and discuss another family situation where the spouse is in denial. The wife has been displaying signs of forgetfulness. The husband is stubborn and is not willing to accept she has a problem and will not take her to a doctor. If you are one of the children, you have no doubt lived many years fearing the wrath of Dad. This guy may be quite opinionated and unwilling to discuss issues; his opinion is the only right opinion. How do you tell Dad that you think mom needs medical help? I know it is simple for me to say that you should take the assertive approach and give Dad an ultimatum to either get help for Mom or you will file endangerment charges. The consequences of this approach may be more than you expected, so let's look at this as potentially the last option. Try to learn why Dad feels there is nothing wrong. Is it because he is truly afraid of losing his wife? Is it because his sister has similar symptoms and is now in a nursing home not remembering anyone? Is it because he does not have the financial resources to provide for her? Is it because he just doesn't know what to do? The first step would be to try to do a process of elimination. Just like with diagnosing Alzheimer's, you may have to determine what it's not. Without pointing to Alzheimer's or dementia, ask Dad if Mom had a heart attack, would he be able to handle the financial burden associated with the illness. If he tells you that is none of your business, you may want to state that if something happens to him, it would become your business. You are not asking how much money he has, but

Due to the nature of this disease, unpopular decisions are sometimes required.

if he has the financial means to handle a serious illness, even if it involved assisted living or nursing home care. If you are still getting nothing, I have heard of a technique that lacks ethics and may violate your parents trust in you. Andrew arranged for his Mom and Dad to be away from the house for a couple of hours. He went into their house to do some investigating. He said he was careful as to keep this a covert mission and leave no evidence behind. Andrew found bank statements, insurance policies, medical information, as well as personal data. He said he wrote down pertinent information and is keeping it in his safe at his house. It is Andrew's plan to only use this information if his father becomes ill and will not be able to care for his mom. Andrew also found some doctor names and contact info for the family attorney. With this new-found information, Andrew was able to eliminate at least one of the reasons as to why dad is being difficult. (Entering into an uninvited property can be considered a criminal offense. You may want to discuss this technique with your attorney first.) As it turned out, Andrew's father became ill and was not able to care for his mom for a period of time. Andrew said he was thankful that he had captured some of the information he needed to best care for his mom. His dad, disappointed as to what Andrew did behind his back, thanked him for his overwhelming compassion.

Helping to educate Dad would be of benefit; however, might I suggest doing this in a more subliminal manner. If you stick literature in front of him, he will likely just throw it away. If you put this book in front of him, you may want to tear out the pages where we learned of Andrew's method of capturing info. You could ask Mom to sit with you and watch "Away From Her," a Julie Christie movie or "The Notebook," featuring James Garner. Chances are that Dad will probably join in. Another idea; try turning to Dad for some fatherly advice. Tell him that a friend at your work is having some difficulty with his mom's dementia. What would Dad suggest in trying to convince your friend to get his mom to the doctor? Maybe even ask Dad if he could go with you to talk with your friend about how to go about helping him and his mom. Explain that your friend's father has passed, and it is just your friend as the sole provider for his mom. Ask if you can rehearse a bit with your dad before the meeting. Of course, a meeting will never occur; your friend's mom suddenly took ill, was hospitalized' and then redirected into a long-term care facility. "Guess the problem solved itself," you would say. During the course of this exercise, you may have developed some insight as to how to turn this back onto your dad.

Often, there is someone that Dad confides in. This may be an old work buddy, the minister, the neighbor, a brother, or as I have also seen, a son-in-law. This person can be used to help convince Dad that he needs to make sure mom is getting proper medical attention. Dad's confidant can even take it as far as guilting Dad into taking action. By telling Dad that sometimes a dementia is hereditary, and he certainly would not want to pass something like this down to the kids. It is important to know what they are dealing with. Dad's comrade could also volunteer to go with Dad to a support group meeting or at least visit with a social worker at the Alzheimer's

Association to get some information. It is important to get Dad talking with someone. Getting Dad in front of someone that has had firsthand experience with dementia can be very helpful in sharing stories, observations, and experiences.

We sometimes realize we must make a change when it finally slaps us in the face. It's great to sit down to a big meal of greasy buffalo wings and onion rings, followed by a burger and fries the next day, and short ribs the following. There is no need to exercise because we have a riding mower, remote controls for everything, and a handicap sticker for our car since we have knee problems. We then wonder why we just woke up in a recovery room after a quadruple heart valve bypass. The next steps will be to diet, exercise, and de-stress. Yes, there were warning signs along the way. The doctor told us we had high blood pressure. After taking your laundry upstairs you were out of breath. We noticed some chest pains, but just did not have time to get it checked out. Death is something that does not wait on us. No matter how healthy of a life you might have lived; I like to say that I have tiptoed through life so I can get to death

> *Our days in life are numbered. The problem is we don't know how many we have left.*

safely; the fact is, we are going to die. What makes it so difficult is that we just do not know when. You must get Dad's attention that Mom needs help. Denial cures nothing. Denial is simply trying to convince your brain to ignore the truth.

Notes:

3. Create a Journal

As a caregiver, we are tired, stressed, unappreciated, depressed, and often malnourished. We forget to do things, miss appointments, forget to ask the doctor about something, and even miss meals because we are too busy. We put our head down and plow forward. We know for every given day, somehow, we have to get from Point A to Point B. We simply get overwhelmed at times and find that our organizational skills get over-tasked. We have to pay bills, run to doctors, make meals, clean and do laundry, dress our loved-ones, bathe them, change them, and manage household and yard maintenance. Writing events on a wall calendar can quickly become your enemy. Your loved-one will look at the scheduled events and continually ask questions or create a barrier for you stating they will not be participating in that scheduled doctor visit. **You have become a single parent caring for an adult child.**

Writing your to-do's down are important and helpful. Managing a calendar will also help to avoid missing events. Taking notes at doctor's visits helps us remember instructions. Before long, you have more notes, calendar entries, and to-dos scattered about that your stress levels have suddenly multiplied. The best way to reduce this stress and better manage your life is to create a journal. Your journal becomes an evolving or organic document. The journal will help control your events, manage notes to and from the doctors, document observations, categorize medications, chart goals, and catalog thoughts. There are various products already on the market such as a personal organizer, day planner, personal analog assistant, personal planner, year planner, bullet journal, or agenda; basically, something that is a small book or binder that is designed to be portable. For computers and smartphones, there are many apps that will also suffice.

Journals help us keep organized so we can quickly recall important information.

Although it would be wise to keep a journal for your own health as well, my objective here is to discuss creating a journal for managing the healthcare of your loved-one. Your journal should be divided into several sections as presented over the next few pages.

Critical Information

Last update:

Full Name:	M/F:
Current Address:	Emergency Contact:
City/State/Zip:	Relationship:
Phone:	Phone:
	Email:
Insurance Provider:	Lives Alone Y/N:
Provider Phone Number:	Smokes/How Much?
Policy/Group #:	Drink Alcohol/How Much?
	Still Driving Y/N:
Recent diagnoses:	Date
	Primary Care Contact:
	Type of physcian:
	Phone:
	Address:
	Email:
Allergies/Symptoms:	
	Pharmacy Contact:
	Phone:
	Address:
Surgeries - Type:	Date
	Internal Devices:
	DNR Y/N:
	PEG Tube Y/N:
	Living Will Y/N:
Recent Testing/Outcome:	Date
	Final Directives:
Blood Pressure ____/____	Glucose Level:	Weight:

Daily Activities

Day of Week:	Date:	General mood:
Sunday		

Make notes based on personal feelings, observations, changes (plus or minus), thoughts, meals...

Day of Week:	Date:	General mood:
Monday		

Make notes based on personal feelings, observations, changes (plus or minus), thoughts, meals...

Day of Week:	Date:	General mood:
Tuesday		

Make notes based on personal feelings, observations, changes (plus or minus), thoughts, meals...

Day of Week:	Date:	General mood:
Wednesday		

Make notes based on personal feelings, observations, changes (plus or minus), thoughts, meals...

Day of Week:	Date:	General mood:
Thursday		

Make notes based on personal feelings, observations, changes (plus or minus), thoughts, meals...

Day of Week:	Date:	General mood:
Friday		

Make notes based on personal feelings, observations, changes (plus or minus), thoughts, meals...

Day of Week:	Date:	General mood:
Saturday		

Make notes based on personal feelings, observations, changes (plus or minus), thoughts, meals...

Page ___ of ___

Care Record (Visits)

Date of Visit	Physician	Office Y/N	Std / Emergency	Purpose/Symptoms			
Plan to discuss (Changes/Observations):							
Instructions from Doctor:							
Next follow-up (date/time):							

Date of Visit	Physician	Office Y/N	Std / Emergency	Purpose/Symptoms			
Plan to discuss (Changes/Observations):							
Instructions from Doctor:							
Next follow-up (date/time):							

Pharmaceutical Record

Date	Calor Code	Medicine/Dosing	Frequency	Purpose	Physician	Pharmacy	Active Y/N	Refill Date

Daily Medication Reminder

Date	Caldr Code		Caldr Code		Caldr Code		Caldr Code		Caldr Code		Caldr Code			Caldr Code			Morning	Lunch	Dinner	Bedtime	Calendar Code				Calendar Code	
*	AM	PM	AM	PM	AM	PM	AM	MID	PM	AM	PM	AM	MID	PM	Morning	Lunch	Dinner	Bedtime	Morning	Lunch	Dinner	Bedtime
Time	Time	Time	Time	Time	Time	Time	Time	Time	Time	Time	Time	Time	Time	Time	Time	Time	Time	Time	Time	Time	Time	Time
1																						
2																						
3																						
4																						
5																						
6																						
7																						
8																						
9																						
10																						
11																						
12																						
13																						
14																						
15																						
16																						
17																						
18																						
19																						
20																						
21																						
22																						
23																						
24																						
25																						
26																						
27																						
28																						
29																						
30																						
31																						

Contact Register of Medical Professionals

Page _____ of _____

Type	Name	Phone	Cell	Email	First Seen
Address				Sepeciality	Still Active Y/N

Type	Name	Phone	Cell	Email	First Seen
Address				Sepeciality	Still Active Y/N

Type	Name	Phone	Cell	Email	First Seen
Address				Sepeciality	Still Active Y/N

Type	Name	Phone	Cell	Email	First Seen
Address				Sepeciality	Still Active Y/N

Type	Name	Phone	Cell	Email	First Seen
Address				Sepeciality	Still Active Y/N

Personal Contacts

Name	Phone	Cell	Email	Relation to Patient
Address				Emergency Y/N
Name	Phone	Cell	Email	Relation to Patient
Address				Emergency Y/N
Name	Phone	Cell	Email	Relation to Patient
Address				Emergency Y/N
Name	Phone	Cell	Email	Relation to Patient
Address				Emergency Y/N
Name	Phone	Cell	Email	Relation to Patient
Address				Emergency Y/N
Name	Phone	Cell	Email	Relation to Patient
Address				Emergency Y/N

Life Story

Include interests and hobbies, work career or profession, achievements and accomplishments, educational specifics, favorite vacation spots, likes and dislikes, and favorite cars owned. Include family details like first name of kids and grandkids, cities lived, anything special or unique with regard to the family members, best friends' names whether alive or not, anniversary, honeymoon location, and favorite restaurant for family events. You can share some stories that you might recall that make your loved-one special. These could be a Purple Heart recipient; have climbed Mt. Everest; restored an antique car; performed in concert with the Rolling Stones; earned a Writers Guild award. Or it could be something very simple as sang in the church choir; would sit on the front porch and read stories to the neighborhood children; as a child would sell lemonade at the corner; or made a skateboard from an old ironing board and rode it down the middle of the street. Ask friends and relatives for their thoughts and memories and add as well.

Name:

Attached to the journal should be a copy of all doctor, hospital, and pharmacy records. You need to include all lab reports and testing results as well. This journal needs to go with you wherever you take your loved-one. You may want to keep a copy at home and one in the car. More about this in the next section.

I have copies of these documents available online for you to download. There is a formatted journal that should be available along with this book at the location where this book was purchased. I also plan to have a smartphone app that will assist you in an all-electronic format. You will be able to take photos of medical documents and attach them to your loved-one's profile.

4. Medical Alignment and Alternative Medicines

If I were to build a house, it would involve more than just a hammer, nails and some boards. To do the job right, I will need an architect, a general contractor, a building supply house, permits, possible zoning modifications, land, and of course some money. I could just let the architect and general contractor decide what type of house they would like to build, or I can get involved and take a proactive role. This is much the same as with healthcare. If we go to a doctor with a particular pain, we are at the mercy of the doctor's diagnosis and our body's time to respond to determine how soon we will feel better.

In considering our aging generation of people, we often see that they are visiting many doctors of varying specialties. They can have one doctor for their heart, another for blood, another for brain health, another for teeth, another for eye care, another for foot problems, and then their general practitioner for routine stuff. Each doctor along the way could prescribe a medicine for a conditional treatment. All these pharmaceuticals can begin fighting one another to where side effects may occur. The GP will normally take control of all the various treatments and medicines, however, that is only if they are provided the information. If a specialist does not provide their treatment log to the GP, the GP will be limited in his ability to oversee your total wellbeing. To compound this, we also assume that when a specialist reports his findings back to our primary care provider that our primary care doctor will actually look at the material before it is filed away in your records.

For these reasons, I profess that it is your responsibility to take control of your health and the health of the loved-one who has entrusted you with her wellbeing. We need to create a three-way relationship or union between the doctor, you, and

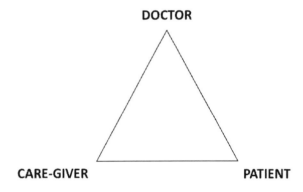

DOCTOR

CARE-GIVER   **PATIENT**

your loved-one. I refer to this as the **care triangle.**

It is important for you to obtain copies of all procedures from all the various doctors for your own records and for the primary care physician's records. The most recent of these documents should be kept in your Wellness Journal. When visiting with doctors, make sure they are aware of the most recent changes made by other health professionals. Then upon completion of your visit, be sure to get a copy of the notes associated with this visit. Some doctors will use dictation devices during the visit. If this is the case with your doctor, make sure to ask the nurse or receptionist to have a copy mailed to you.

Although I say you need to adhere to this care triangle, there may be times when your primary care physician may have a different idea or just does not have the time to give the attention you feel is necessary. There are times when you go to visit a doctor and are seen by a physician assistant. There may be times when the doctor is just so busy they are in and out of the examination room faster than the amount of time it takes to realize that burner is still hot and to remove your hand.

Doctors have to complete multiple years of college plus additional years of residency. We walk into their offices and see all these certificates on the walls. This makes us feel intimidated. We tend to feel an inward fear when meeting with them. My father said that he is not as much interested in seeing all the certificates as he is interested in seeing their report cards. He would say that with his luck, the very reason he was at the doctor was the class in which the doctor received a failing grade. We need to remember that doctors are people too. They have children, some have grandchildren. They go to the ballpark, picnics, and shop at many of the same stores where we shop. You may sit next to a doctor at church, you may be in an elevator at the department store with a doctor, why even sitting in the waiting room at the muffler repair center you could be sitting with two or three doctors, and even at your favorite sports event you will find many.

If we were standing in line at a grocery store behind a man that is simply not placing his groceries on the conveyor at the speed we would like to see, our natural tendency is to be judgmental of this guy and critique every single item he places in front of the cashier. If when paying, the cashier addresses him as doctor, we would then look back at him and say to our self, "Wow, I didn't see that one coming." Just one day prior, we were feeling intimidated to be in front of our doctor, to where we then become the critic of what we believe is a self-centered, inconsiderate person.

There are reasons why doctors may give you the impression they either do not have enough time for you or act as if they do not care. Without arguing whether it is right or wrong, the more patients the doctor sees in a given day is indirectly proportional to how much time he spends with you. Of course, we want the doctor to give us as much time as we feel is needed. However, due to insurance company restrictions, physician fees are somewhat controlled in the US. Becoming a doctor is a tremendously expensive profession to choose. We need doctors and they deserve to be paid. It is entirely up to the doctor to determine his specialty, how many patients he would like to see in a given day, and how much time he feels is needed per patient.

We want the doctor to spend enough time to listen to us and answer our questions. There is nothing wrong with that and that is what the doctors want as well. Unfortunately, some patients can be a little long-winded in their dissertation to the doctor. When Katherine tells her doctor, "Well we were at church last Sunday, we went to the early service because the children were doing a special program, and our granddaughter, Melissa, the youngest one, is part of the youth choir so we did not want to miss it. She has such a lovely voice and it is such a joy to see these kids perform; well after the service we stopped for lunch at Bob Evans, you know the new one they just built right off the highway there across from the old Wellston estate. It was so sad to see them tear that down only to build a shopping center. Who needs another shopping center? Half of it is still vacant! So, as we were leaving,

Keys factors in maintaining a successful relationship with your doctor: honesty, openness, mutual respect, and trust.

and I was getting into the car, and I keep telling Bob, my husband, that we need to get rid of that old thing and get something with bigger doors, was when I scraped my ear on that metal strip that goes across the top of the door frame, that shiny thing that keeps the water from going down over the windows when it is raining." Now if everyone that visited that doctor that day had a similar story just to say that they scraped their ear on a car door frame, the doctor would have to send people home untreated.

Of course, there are also those that are so intimidated by the doctor that they are afraid to say anything. Sometimes it's like we do not want the doctor to know about that mole because it is simply embarrassing; it is so ugly and keeps growing. Needless to say, not a good decision! Believe me, I understand. I have done just that, thinking it will be gone by my next visit. But, of course, there I am back within another week or two and now we are talking about the thing I didn't want to tell him about prior. The doctor is your confidant. He is the one you can share all your health secrets with and not be judged. The doctor may tell you to stop doing something that could be harmful, and for the most part, his advice will be in your best interest. If for any reason, the doctor is anything less than professional, you should first tell him of your concern. If the action continues, he can be reported, or you can take your business elsewhere.

If you are in the doctor's examination room and you feel the doctor is not giving you adequate time, the proper things to do would be either to ask the doctor if this time is not the best for a conversation on this subject, or when should you return? Another option is to simply stand between the doctor and the door. I have never heard of a doctor shoving a patient out of the way just to get out of the room. If you choose this tactic, I would suggest being to the point and professional. You just might need another appointment; if you know what I am saying…

Due to the complexity of the disease, other undiagnosed conditions, the doctor's due diligence, the information shared with the medical professionals, possible drug interactions/side-effects, and the individuals body chemistry; the doctor may not always be right in his findings. There are so many other things that masks themselves to look like dementia. A thyroid imbalance, low B12 levels (also Vitamin D, Folic Acid, and Magnesium), medication interactions, depression, dehydration, a urinary tract infection, low blood oxygen levels, blood infection, alcoholism, antihistamines, and a concussion can all appear as or contribute to the appearance of dementia. During the preliminary medical exams, most of these areas may not be tested or discussed. Symptoms can continue indefinitely until you either specifically ask for these tests or evaluations or come upon a doctor that has the time to spend reviewing these areas. Most of the items I just mentioned can be corrected and thereby restoring the patient's memory skills.

Maggie, a middle-age daughter, attended one of my support group sessions and stated that her mom is not doing well, in fact, they called in hospice care. I asked her to explain more. Maggie said that her mom was always very meticulous in her appearance. At the assisted living facility, she would never be seen outside of her room without full make-up, her hair appearing as if it was just cut and styled, and her dress and shoes appearing as if she was at the least on her way to a fine dining event. She was very engaging with her table-mates in the dining area. All the other women were very complimentary of the mom when talking with Maggie. The daughter said that it seemed her mom had a rather quick decline to where she would not even want to get out of bed. When her mom would go to the dining area, she needed to be directed to her table because she did not recognize her table buddies. Soon, the mom would not leave her room.

I began asking some questions about her mom's general health, outside of the dementia. I asked about blood tests, B12 levels, and recent changes in her diet and activities. Maggie said the doctor said the blood levels were fine and could not identify any changes that has recently occurred. I asked if her mom has had her thyroid tested. Maggie said she thought it was tested via her mom's doctor. I explained a bit about the function of the thyroid and why she may want to consider having a more thorough blood test performed. A few weeks later, Maggie attended another group session. She said she took her mom to a thyroid specialist in town and found that via a thyroid panel, her mom's thyroid was not functioning properly, so the doctor prescribed some necessary medication. Maggie was there to report that her mom is now going back to the dining room and sitting with her buddies. She is putting on her make-up, doing her hair, and dressing herself as lovely as always. It was an amazing example of how we sometimes need to be the patient advocate for our loved-one.

The thyroid is a critical part of our pituitary system. The thyroid regulates many of the body's processes, such as metabolism, energy generation, and mood. A body's heart rate and digestive functions, muscle control, and brain development are the functions of the thyroid. About 17% of women over 60 will experience some form of Hypothyroidism. The American Thyroid Association suggests the following:

What do the following patients over the age of 60 years have in common?

1. *A 72-year-old woman with "fluttering of the heart" and vague chest discomfort on climbing stairs*
2. *An 80-year-old man with severe constipation who falls asleep often*

3. A 65-year-old woman who has lost strength in her legs, causing difficulty in climbing stairs; she has recently lost 15 lbs. in spite of a very good appetite
4. A 75-year-old woman who has developed difficulty swallowing and a dry cough, accompanied by hoarseness, weight gain, and dry, itchy skin
5. A 78-year-old man with hearing loss
6. An 84-year-old woman in whom a hand tremor has caused her to give up favorite activities. She is so depressed that she will not eat, and she has lost 12 lbs. in the last 4 months.

All of these patients have abnormal function of their thyroid glands. Patients 1, 3 and 6 have hyperthyroidism, that is, excessive production of thyroid hormone by their thyroid glands. Patients 2, 4 and 5 have hypothyroidism, or reduced production of thyroid hormone. While some of the symptoms of hyperthyroidism and hypothyroidism are similar to those in younger patients, it is not uncommon for both hyperthyroidism and hypothyroidism to manifest in subtle ways in older patients, often masquerading as diseases of the bowel or heart or a disorder of the nervous system. An important clue to the presence of thyroid disease in an elderly patient is a history of thyroid disease in another close family member such as a brother, sister or child of the patient.

In particular, if there is a family history of thyroid disease or suspicion of such, it would be advisable to bring this to the attention of a physician.

Vitamin B12 is called "the most important nutrient we don't think about." The reason is that B12 is critical to our clarity. This is a nutrient that can be stored in our body, different from most others. If something causes our B12 level to deplete below 300 ng/L, we are likely to experience weakness, fatigue, irritability, and memory loss. B12 is found in animal foods and some fortified cereals. The vitamin is absorbed into the bloodstream via the stomach. As we age, we are ingesting items that effect how food and minerals are absorbed. Aspirin, antacids, and proton-pump inhibitors like omeprazole, decrease stomach acids that are needed to extract necessary proteins, vitamin B12, and calcium. A common diabetes medication can do the same as well. This reduction in B12 can also cause our DNA to not replicate properly, meaning this deficiency can mimic all the effects of aging.

> *Vitamin B12 – the most important nutrient we never think about.*

Fortunately, when caught in time, we can begin receiving B12 injections to bring our levels back to the proper state. Following, a maintenance dose administered by the physician will likely be needed to insure our B12 level remains in a safe zone.

My friend, Mark, was having some kidney stone problems. His urologist told him that he wants to do a full metabolic panel on him in order to determine a baseline for evaluation. The metabolic panel is a blood evaluation that measures a gambit of key components within our body. This includes uric acid, electrolytes, calcium, phosphorus, etc. From this initial evaluation, a second test can be performed a few months later to help determine what may be causing a stone to form. The problem was that Mark was taking a form of omeprazole and a handful of vitamins daily. The urologist told him to stop taking all vitamins and aspirin-based products. After a few weeks, the baseline test was performed. The mistake was that Mark should have had the baseline metabolic panel performed when he was taking all the vitamins because when the second test was done, there was no change from the baseline. It was likely, something associated with the vitamins that was playing a part in the formation of the stones. I believe, the second mistake this urologist made was in overlooking the need for the B12 that was provided via a supplement. Over the next several months, Mark began showing a lack of energy and seemed to have some issue in remembering names and times. I brought this change in personality to his attention. He went to his family doctor for a physical. A B12 blood analysis indicated that his B12 levels had dropped to a questionable level. Following some B12 injections, Mark is back to his old self.

Via my support group, I experienced several similar stories regarding severely low B12 levels and how it was affecting love-ones. Outside of diabetes, changes in diet or acid-reducing medications are why older people may experience a reduction in B12 levels.

Coming on the scene recently is the connection of a Vitamin D deficiency and dementia. Studies are beginning to show a relationship with low Vitamin D levels resulting in a quicker decline in memory and cognitive abilities. This is particularly due to Vitamin D's role in strengthening our immune system. Your loved-one

The sunshine vitamin - Those that stay out of the sun, suffer from milk allergies, or are on a strict vegan diet, may be at risk of a Vitamin D deficiency.

may not want to go outside due to incontinence, lack of interest, or changes in habits. According to research, many are deficient of Vitamin D. The bulk of our daily intake of Vitamin D comes from the sun. Cloudy days, smog, sunscreen, and length of daylight play a role in reducing our daily intake. Indoors, behind a window, all the Vitamin D producing UV rays are blocked. Few foods provide this valuable vitamin with exception of Cod liver oil, Swordfish, and Salmon. Otherwise, we rely on "fortified with Vitamin D" foods like orange juice, milk, and yogurt. Certainly, a vitamin supplement of Vitamin D can help offset this shortfall. Too much of a good thing can also be bad. I urge you to consult your physician. You should be cautious of toxicity caused by too much Vitamin D and possible interactions with medications or steroids.

A magical potion that most of us tend to overlook is water. Our bodies average around 57% - 60% water. So, it is not likely we will drown from drinking too much water. When we lose only 2% of our body's water, we begin to feel thirsty. By that time, we have already been affected by mental and physical impairments. The water in the brain is 73%. A minor drop in hydrogenation can have life-threatening effects. Water carries oxygen and nutrients to our cells. It is the principal solvent in the body. Water is the transport agent that insulates, lubricates, metabolizes, flushes, and regulates.

The trouble with water? When we drink it, we then have to pee it out. What a waste of time, and effort. It is easier to not drink water and just continue with life. We are then not interrupted with that nagging bladder pain and need to make time to go to the bathroom. All too often, this becomes a lifestyle for the elderly. It is too far to walk to the bathroom. It is too difficult to get up out of the chair. There is no place to go when out on a walk or grocery shopping. The bathroom process is too difficult or takes too long. So, what happens? They make a psychological choice to skip the water. Before long, they get dizzy, fall, and are transported to the hospital where the first thing the medics will do is start them on fluids.

Signs of mild to moderate dehydration include dry mouth, headache, bad breath, mood changes, muscle cramps, darker urine, thirst, fatigue, lightheadedness, and cloudy thinking. Severe dehydration indicators are rapid breathing, extreme thirst, low blood pressure, no urination, severe dizziness, rapid heartbeat, no skin moisture, and unconsciousness.

It can be very difficult at times to get your loved-one to keep drinking water when they refuse to do so. Dehydration is one of the leading reasons why a senior will visit an emergency room. As we age, it becomes increasingly more difficult for our bodies to retain water. Between not remembering to drink water and various medications that act as diuretics, our bodies actually need more water and electrolytes. And don't get me started on electrolytes.

Ok, you just did. The aging process takes its toll on our kidneys. Our kidneys play a key role in managing the electrolytes in our body. An imbalance in electrolytes can surface as an irregular heartbeat, weakness, *Dehydration is one of the leading reasons why a senior will visit an emergency room.* twitching, confusion, numbness, excessive tiredness, convulsions and muscle spasms. Causes such as prolonged periods of vomiting or diarrhea, severe dehydration, congestive heart failure, diuretics, and aging, play significant factors in effecting the healthy levels of magnesium, sodium, potassium, bicarbonate, chloride, phosphate, and calcium; all electrolytes within our body. Your physician can help you determine if any of these levels may need adjusted.

Okay, you get it, more water; but how? Sometimes adding flavors to water will help, such as adding some juice, or squeezing an orange or lemon into the water. Maybe add a garnish. This can make drinking water look more interesting while making them feel like the elite. Water comes in various varieties, like decaffeinated coffee or tea, broths, popsicles, and crushed ice beverages like smoothies. Another method of increasing the water intake comes from cucumbers which have a 96% water content, iceberg lettuce, celery, radishes, tomatoes, bell peppers, grapes, oranges, cauliflower, watermelon, spinach, strawberries, broccoli, grapefruit, and cantaloupe are all great sources of water and vital nutrients as well. Get the blender out, add some ice, and you have a pretty yummy drink.

There are ways of consuming water that may not be in your loved-ones best interest. This includes caffeinated coffee and tea, water or ice in alcoholic beverages, water that has been sitting for too long, water from a plastic container that has been exposed to excessive heat, caffeinated colas, flavored water with artificial sweeteners and additives, and from containers that have not been cleaned regularly.

Another concern is that your father might be willing to drink, but just does not remember how to do so. Or he knows he will have to go to the bathroom where he has difficulty in maneuvering through the process. His mind may be trying to protect him from this difficult task by telling him not to drink. Eyesight, depth of field, and grip can also be interfering with willingness to drink. When he reaches out for the glass, does he knock it over or have difficulty in lifting or holding the bottle? Or, maybe he just does not remember it is there and/or has not become thirsty. Often times, an Alzheimer's patient's body does not tell him what he needs or how he feels.

One other topic I would like to quickly touch on in this section is the urinary tract infection, or UTI. A UTI is a bacterial infection, more common in women, that can be a real nuisance for a dementia patient. Without going into the causes of the UTI for either men or women, let's discuss how this nasty infection can affect the body and mind. The frequent trips to the bathroom or the use of the disposable underwear (due to all the water I just told you was important,) you may have to deal with a possible side effect as a result. The UTI can cause an intense urge to urinate, but nothing comes out; can cause a severe burning feeling when urinating; a dark color or odor can result; and a fever or chills can be noticed. A UTI can also cause a cognitive change in your loved-one. This could be seen as a noticeable increase in confusion, agitation, or withdrawal. One day your wife may act semi-normal and the next she is irritated and cannot remember who you are to her. Interestingly, once the UTI is treated and cleared, she is back to semi-normal state.

I was given an opportunity to view a test at a nursing home where they gave several patients a picture of a grandfather clock and asked them to draw the grandfather clock on another piece of paper. Most did an awesome job in drawing the clock. As some of these patients were diagnosed with a UTI, the same "test" was put in front of them. The drawings that these folks drew were mostly undetectable to be a clock. After the UTI had cleared, the patients were retested. There was that awesome clock drawing again, properly shaped, with the round face and hands.

5. Change Your Thinking

"Perception is reality." That is a quote that every sales person needs to understand in order to be successful. What the customer perceives becomes that customer's reality. If the customer perceives the salesman to be unknowledgeable on a particular topic, does it make the customer wrong? It is the opinion of the customer. Opinions can be changed and therefore if this sales person wants to turn this prospect into a customer, he must change this person's opinion or perception.

If your son were to approach you and tell you he doesn't like school, does it make him wrong? No, it is simply his opinion. His reality of school is riddled with challenges that need to be dealt with in order to change his perception. He may be faced with a bully, he may have girlfriend problems, or he could be struggling with a subject. In any case, as a parent, we need to understand why his perception of school is distorted. It is our job to offer help or correction.

Your loved-one is living in her own reality. As her memory becomes disassociated with actual reality, we have to do one of two things; we have to retrain or accept. Notice I did not say WHO needs retrained. If your loved-one makes a comment about the yellow paint on the walls and the color is actually green, does it make him wrong? Keep in mind he learned the color yellow when he was two years old. By telling him the walls are green, you are telling him he has been wrong all his life. Imagine how you would feel if someone told you something you believed to be true for 80 years is now wrong. It is their perception. If we choose to retrain them, by telling them the wall is green, we often start an argument. Guess who always wins the argument with an Alzheimer's patient? If you think it is you, I urge you to go back to the beginning of this book and reread everything back to this point. Go ahead. I will wait for you right here.

We have to retrain ourselves. We have to understand that their reality becomes quite a bit different from our reality. In the example just given, wouldn't it be much better to just agree with their comment about the yellow walls. In the end, is it the color of the walls or the color of the shirt or the color of the pill that really matters?

To better understand what is occurring let's look at the brain's memory as an onion. Each layer of the onion represents a time in our life. The most recent occurrences reside on the outermost layer while the deep-rooted memories reside in the core. As a dementia patient progresses through the disease, the layers of the onion begin peeling off. Remembering what they had for lunch or who came to visit cannot be retained because that layer is now gone. There is nothing there to store those thoughts. Eventually, more and more layers begin falling off to where conversations are then centered around a time many years ago. I often refer to this as "time travel."

As they travel back in time, their reality changes. This creates confusion for them because what they are seeing does not gel with what they perceive. A mention of, "I want to go home," when we know mom is at home, where in fact mom is referring to her childhood home and not this home where she lived for the past 38 years. Again, we tell her, you are at home. Of course, this only adds to the confusion. Their perception of home may be somewhere they lived prior or that of a place visited or viewed on a television show. All is based on the layers of the onion as to where they are in time. I moved my mother into a full-care facility from a nearby apartment. I had not completed the move and asked her if she wanted to help. She lived in this apartment for nearly a year. Upon entering the apartment from having not been in it for just over a week, she commented on how beautiful this apartment was to her and asked who lives here. I took her to her closet to ask what clothes she would like to take with her to her "new home." In opening the doors, she said, "These clothes are so lovely, whose are they?" I told her that they were her clothes. Her comment to me, "Don't be silly."

You as the male spouse may initially "become" a brother or a boyfriend to your wife. Eventually, you may "become" her father. Although reality changes for them, their perception of what they are witnessing is adjusted by recent familiarity. To frame it differently, you are the male figure to where there is an inner attachment, one she cannot identify, and therefore you now must "become" her father. Michael, an older gentleman that attended my support group was approached by his wife; she said, "Now tell me again, who are you?" He said, "Honey, I am your husband." To which she replied, "Why on earth would I be married to an old man like you?" You can see that she had travelled back in time to where her reality was placing her into her younger years.

> As a "time traveler" travels back in time, today never happened. Anything more current that their perceived reality has never existed.

Another husband, Sam, reported to me that his wife referred to him as her boyfriend, a handyman, once in a while her husband, and a complete stranger. Finally, after Sam was standing in his living room for the second time in handcuffs placed by the local police following a 911 call about a stranger in her house, Sam was able to explain to the police that his wife is suffering from dementia. Sam said, look at the mantle above the fireplace, that is my picture there with my wife. That is not what a home invader does. Sam then learned that he had to role play with his wife. Based on how she would address him, he would have to fall into that role in order to minimize her confusion. I guess you can say he had to become a magician. He would change roles almost instantly to follow her lead. Sam had to adapt in order to maintain peace and manage a quality of life for his wife.

Carla, a woman living with her husband effected with dementia was asked every night if she left the door unlocked so Dad can get in. Terry, a middle age daughter would get a call from her mom every night asking if the mom's children had a ride home. Nancy, a female patient at the full care facility where my mother lived, would ask everyone she saw if they knew how to find her bus pass. She cannot get home without her bus pass. The stories go on and on. Learning how to react to these events will determine if we calm or agitate. I would tell Nancy that I found her bus pass and will give it to her before I leave. Her face would light up and on one occasion, gave me a big hug in gratitude.

We like to show grandma pictures of the grandkids. We point to each of them in the photo and name them by name. Grandma usually replies, "What a beautiful bunch of children, now tell me again, who do they belong to?" You might as well be showing her a framed photo you just purchased at Walmart. Even showing her current photos of herself may often create confusion. If her image of herself is of many years earlier, why does that person in the photo look so old? One fellow told me that his wife would spend hours looking into a mirror talking to the older woman in the reflection.

As time travel occurs, events that have taken place in the "future" may become grounds for contention. If your mother happens to be one of these time travelers and she asks, "When will your father be home?" and your father passed away 15 years ago; you may have a mess on your hands if you do not answer her properly. If you say, "Mom, Dad is dead." Imagine how you would feel if you found out suddenly that your soul mate is dead? Not to mention when you tell her, "Yeah, he died 15 years ago." Every emotion known to mankind could suddenly pass in front of you. I heard a story once where the mom asked the daughter about when the father would be home. The daughter replied, "Mom, dad died two years ago." The mom looking sternly at the daughter said, "Well, that explains a lot!"

You have heard about the book, "Men are from Mars, Women are from Venus" by John Gray, Ph.D. In the book, we learn that men and women communicate differently, have a different set of values, and experience emotions differently. Men want to fix things when women only want to be listened to. I am here to profess that Alzheimer's patients are from the planet Neptune. Mars and Venus are our neighboring planets. Neptune is "currently" our farthest planet and furthest away from the Sun. We know the least about Neptune. So, if we were to think of our loved-ones, stricken with some form of dementia, being from the planet Neptune, you can see we would have to change our thinking to better understand theirs. At times, we need to actually go onto their planet, if that were possible, to realize why they are displaying strange behavior or saying crazy stuff. **We tend to spend all our time trying to bring**

them back into our world. In our world they are now an alien. **We must get into their world if we truly want to help.**

As this onion begins to peel back, so too are the connections with other layers. Word associations become disconnected. You may offer gravy for their mashed potatoes and they think you are offering car oil. Have you noticed recently when you and dad go out to eat, he often points to pictures on the menu. You think to yourself that this is not what he normally orders, but why create a problem. It is a good idea to offer to order for him or mention to him what you two usually order when coming to this restaurant and would he like the same again. Likely, you will have put dad at ease and the ordering process is behind you so now you can spend quality time with your father.

> *We must get into their world. Our world does not exist to them.*

As changes occur with the dementia patient's cognitive skills, behavioral problems may occur. The patient can experience:

- Irritability (easily agitated)
- Anxiety (crying, loving, anxious)

- Depression (question their existence or threats to harm themselves)
- Sleep disturbances
- Physical or verbal outbursts
- Emotional distress
- Restlessness, pacing, shredding paper or tissues and yelling
- Delusions (firmly held belief in things that are not real)
- Hallucinations (seeing, hearing, or feeling things that are not there.)

These symptoms are likely tied to the continued degeneration of the brain cells, other factors can contribute such as side effects from medications and other illnesses. When exposed to one of these behaviors from your loved-one, keep calm, try to distract their attention away from what is causing their distress, and give them a hug. By telling them that what they experienced is not real, may create more of the same, or add to their confusion and frustration. In any case, each of these behavioral topics are real to them at the time and need managed properly.

Some of the above listed behavioral items can occur based on what your loved-one is witnessing coming from you. Let's face it, this is a long, bumpy road. We get frustrated, cry, and sometimes loose our temper and lash out, maybe not at them but at someone or something. These actions may be copied or mimicked by our loved-one. Hallucinations are part of their reality. My mom would tell me there was a man looking in her window. Each day, she would say the same thing. The interesting factor was that she lived on the third floor. On another occasion, we were watching a show when a news blurb interrupted. Bill Clinton was the President at the time. My mom said, "That man looks very familiar, I think I used to date him." I had no words. She once asked me who the little girl was laying on the floor. It was my jacket that I set there when I came in to visit.

In each of these examples, she truly believed her reality. Lana told me that her mom would wake up at night and come over to her bedroom and tell Lana there was a man in her bedroom. Lana would get up, turn the lights on, and walk her mom back to bed. This went on sometimes a couple of times a night. Finally, Lana decided to "catch the perpetrator". Lana sat in her mom's bedroom with her mom sleeping and in the dark. It was then that she saw a dark shadow on the wall in the form of a man. It was from the street light reflecting upon her mother's drape. Lana adjusted the drape and it was off to dreamland. In this case, light became the culprit in creating a shadow. In most instances, by adding more light to a room the hallucinations are reduced. Please, take these "visions" seriously. If a hallucination occurs that causes your husband to become aggressive in some fashion, there is a chance you may be on the morning news.

Be sure to document each of these odd behaviors with whatever circumstances occurred prior. Share these findings with the physician. If behaviors become harmful to you or to your loved-one, medication may become necessary.

Notes:

6. Initiate a Durable Power of Attorney

Wikipedia describes a Power of Attorney (POA) or letter of attorney as "a written authorization to represent or act on another's behalf in private affairs, business, or some other legal matter." The person authorizing the other to act is the principal, grantor, or donor. It goes on to say, another form is a specific type of power of attorney or health care proxy, in which the person authorizes someone (an agent) to make decisions on their behalf when they are incapacitated. People are often encouraged to complete both documents to provide comprehensive guidance regarding their care, although they may be combined into a single form. These documents are critical when providing care for another that is not capable of making rational, logical decisions.

A characteristic of Alzheimer's Disease can cause the patient to become very generous with their money. They can lose the sense of value such as the monetary difference between $10 and $100. Phone calls requesting donations, mailers asking for help for charities, and door-to-door solicitors can all become their best friends. I have seen where a man diagnosed with Alzheimer's agreed to replace all his windows and siding simply because a young aggressive sales person knocked on his door and convinced him how much nicer the house would look and feel if he spent over $20,000. Fortunately, this man's son was able to put a stop to the purchase just in the nick of time.

From a health perspective, how many times have you asked your affected loved-one how they are feeling, and their response is, "Couldn't be better." I had to take my mother to the ER one evening after learning she had fallen and severely hurt her wrist. As she was being seen by the ER doctor, he asked why she had come to see him. My mom responded that she had no idea as to why she was there and felt perfectly fine. About an hour later, we left with a cast on her lower arm and hand.

Assigning another individual to assist in managing financial and legal matters helps avoid serious disasters. Assigning someone to oversee the individual's healthcare assures the patient is being monitored via their trusted advocate.

The Durable Power of Attorney (DPA) is designed to provide the power of attorney's authority beyond the period of when the principal becomes incapacitated. Once the patient is diseased, the DPA terminates. It is only a legal authority while the person is alive. Another characteristic for Alzheimer's Disease is just the opposite of generosity, it is their fear that they have no money or becoming overly protective of their money. With either behavioral symptom, the management of the money becomes critical. Your husband can foolishly spend all the money to where you have nothing. And to the opposite, bills may need paid, but he will not sign the checks. Regardless of how much energy you expel in trying to convince him not to worry about the money, your efforts will get you nowhere; unless of course you want to make him extremely irritated. By initiating the DPA, you can interact with the bank, the utility company, a credit card company, the financial planner; essentially, anyone or anything that has to do with finances or contracts.

The difficult part is often getting the husband to sign his financial rights over to you. Men are typically more difficult, by nature, to convince to initiate a DPA than a woman. In some cases, the husband or dad can become so obstinate that you may have to begin legal procedures in order to get

> *The POA can be granted limited rights if chosen by the principal. The POA is to act in the best interest of the person to which the POA applies.*

a DPA in place. I have seen where such action forced the court to appoint the POA, which often becomes a court appointed attorney. Hopefully, your situation is much simpler. Of course, the best way to initiate the DPA is via the elder law attorney. The attorney can also prepare the Healthcare Proxy, the Living Will, DNR documents, and the Last Will in Testament that could include the naming of the executor of the Will (if needed).

One very important step: All of this <u>must</u> be done prior to any authority's declaration of cognitive impairment. Simply stated, if your loved-one has been identified to have a mental impairment, such as dementia, their signing of a legal document is non-binding and can be

You can only sign a power of attorney if legally competent to do so.

contested by the court or other family members; for the most part, anyone that feels they should have a say as to how a contract is managed or how money might be distributed. The term "authority" would mean someone qualified to render an accurate medical opinion or diagnosis. In one situation that I recall, Harold, a widower, had been declared cognitively impaired via his doctor. Soon afterwards, Harold fell in love with Elizabeth and they were married. Because Harold began making some questionable financial decisions, his new bride began to take over that role. A few months passed when one of Harold's children asked about a property that Dad owns. Elizabeth told him that due to his inability to make rational decisions, she had the property transferred into her name and that the son would now have no claim to it. Needless to say, this case was taken to court where the judge ruled the marriage was not legal since Harold was diagnosed cognitively impaired and could not enter into a legal contract; such as a marriage. Fortunate, I guess for Elizabeth, she was able to avoid fraud charges in having known that he was cognitively impaired. The moral to the story; in the US, if a doctor or court appointed authority declares an individual has a cognitive impairment, that individual cannot legally enter into a contract. To the earlier example of the window sales person, had the windows been installed, his next stop could have been to court to seek a financial judgement.

If your loved-one is no longer legally permitted to sign the DPA, the only legal option or recourse is to have a guardianship process filed with the court. The court appointed guardian is then responsible to manage the financial matters and possibly the healthcare decisions associated with the person declared mentally incapacitated. This option can come at a steep price.

The DPA for healthcare, also known as health care proxy, is much like the financial DPA with the exception that this is specific for healthcare needs. It allows an entrusted person to become involved with your healthcare decision making. It gives them the authority to speak for you. This individual is granted access to all of your medical information. The patient allows for full disclosure of records, procedures, tests, recommendations, pharmaceuticals, and treatments as permitted by their local laws. This document can allow for the redirection of care to the extent of final life preparations. A healthcare DPA can be rescinded by the patient at any time. If the patient's cognitive skills have been determined to be impaired, a court order will likely be the only way the healthcare DPA can be rescinded or redirected.

As with the financial POA, there can be other family members or friends that may not agree that you should have been entrusted with this decision-making authority. At times, other family members may feel there is nothing wrong with Mom and therefore, the DPA is not needed. At times, others will comment that you are not qualified to work in Mom's best interest. And, there will be times when

Mom may argue with you on the purpose of these DPA documents and deny signing anything of the such. Your job will be met with challenges. You will want to step aside and suggest someone else manages Mom's care. Often you will find that no one else will want to do it. They would just prefer to complain that you are not doing a good job at it.

The US Health Insurance Portability and Accountability Act of 1996 (HIPAA) was established to protect the privacy and security of medical information. This has nothing to do with the quality of care provided or needed for a patient. HIPAA is only for the protection of information associated with an individual's medical information, whether oral, written, or electronic. Interestingly, this actually only applies to the medical providers and healthcare insurance providers. There is a list of others that can have access to this information without your approval...don't get me started on that one.

In most situations, as the DPA proxy (holder), you have all the same access to the medical information as would the patient. You may have to provide copies of your DPA to the multiple healthcare providers, they may be stubborn in sharing information, but rest assured you will be able to have access to this information.

Ron, a caregiver, came to me to ask, "When I dropped my wife off at the doctor's office entrance, my wife went on inside while I was parking the car. When I got inside, the staff had already taken my wife back to visit with the doctor. I asked if I can go back and was told that she is with the doctor now and will be out in just a minute." He continued, "When she came out, I was called over to pay for the exam. I noticed she was holding some written prescriptions. I paid, we left." Ron said, "On the way home, I asked my wife about the visit with the doctor. She said that the doctor said everything was fine. I asked why she received the prescriptions and when is she supposed to take the medication." "My wife said she did not remember, that they are probably nothing important." Now here is when this story gets crazy, Ron continued, "So when I got home, I called the doctor's office to ask about the prescriptions and what notes the doctor had collected. The receptionist told me that she cannot share any information about my wife since I was not part of the visit with the doctor."

> As the POA for your husband, always carry a copy of the DPA with you.

Ron asked what I would recommend. The next day Ron went to the doctor's office with his wife at his side. When greeted at the receptionist's window, he was asked how she can help. Ron said, "My wife had a visit with the doctor yesterday and I was not given permission to be with her during her time with the doctor. I called you soon after and you would not share any information with me about the visit or her care. So, I am leaving her here with you so you and your staff can take care of her." He turned and started walking away; his wife just stayed at the receptionist's window. Needless to say, Ron got the information he needed. The nurse gave Ron the proper forms to sign allowing him access to his wife's information, and a very big apology once they realized the difficulty they caused for this man in just trying to care for his wife.

Ron could have been submissive and let the system control him. He chose to take the initiative to be proactive in order to best provide the quality of life that his wife so deserves. This is only another example of why we as caregivers have to be proactive.

7. Develop a Financial Plan

If I had a nickel for every time my wife has told me that we need a Financial Plan, well, I guess I would not need a Financial Plan. Alzheimer's can be an extremely expensive disease. Most of us do not have an endless supply of money, so we need to approach this topic using as much good judgement as possible.

If money were of no issue, our choices for caregiving become ala carte. We can hire a staff of providers that is capable of 24-hour care, while keeping Mom in her own home. When more skilled or professional attention is needed, a private ambulance can be hired for transport to the proper provider. Depending on where you live, some medical professionals can come to her at her home. This care can, no doubt, be the best for the patient as long as they interact well with the staff and mom does not become combative to the point where it becomes difficult to find willing staff.

For the rest of us, we need to determine how we can provide care for Dad on a budget. The choices are to hire an elder law attorney or visit your local US Medicaid office and follow their instruction to the best of your ability.

Why an elder law attorney versus one that specializes in other areas? Tax laws are always changing. Trusts, life insurance, property ownership, stocks and pension funds, allowable disbursements, and survivor assets as they pertain to the senior citizen fall under the definition of the elder law attorney. It is like hiring a podiatrist to remove your wisdom teeth. Does the podiatrist kinda know the general procedure; maybe. Do I want the person inside of my mouth to be an expert in his field: oh yeah! Hence the need for the elder law attorney. They are simply the best source to help you to figure out what to do with your assets in order to provide quality care for your loved-one.

> **Never throw away documents relating to financial, medical, or government-issued material.**

Some elder law attorneys work on an upfront fee basis, while others are hourly. Regardless, each will get you to the end goal. If laws change or an unforeseen fluctuation to your assets suddenly occurs, the attorney that you have under contract may make the changes to your program at no additional cost. A pay-as-you-go attorney may require another sum of money to make the corrections for you. As with most contract help, it is advised to seek referrals.

Ask your friends, ask your physician, and ask your local Alzheimer's Association for names of elder law attorneys in your area. You may be shocked when you see their fees. However, based on your specific financial condition, this may be a small price to pay for peace of mind.

If you are a dependent or joint (spouse or disabled child) with the loved-one, you still need to live. Nearly all states have provisions that provide a financial means for the direct survivor. You still need a place to live, food to eat, and transportation. As a result, these provisions are factored into the plan recommended by your elder law attorney. It is important to disclose as much as possible to your chosen attorney.

A failure in the legal system in the US is labeled the Medicaid Divorce. This process may qualify an individual for Medicaid to pay for nursing home expenses, however, it is a dissolution of the marriage. This dissolution removes the well spouse from pensions, Supplemental Security Income, and veteran benefits. Courts are to be cautious that the divorce is not a means of getting around regulations of the Medicaid system. Sadly, there are couples that have been in love with each other for 50+ years and their attorney is recommending a Medicaid Divorce as an alternative. Worse yet, the well spouse looks at this as their only alternative, however saying that this breaks their heart is stating it lightly.

If attorney fees are not something you can afford, or you believe the assets are such that Medicaid is in the very near future; you can consider your local Legal Aid Society office for assistance, your church, or possibly going at it on your own. This method is certainly not the easiest of your options, but on the other hand, may be your only option. As soon and early as possible, you will need to meet with your local Medicaid office. You will learn from them exactly what is and will be needed in order to qualify for Medicaid. This generally includes a pile of documents, proofs of identification, financial and medical histories of possibly up to 7 – 10 years back, an inventory of all assets including life insurance(s), CD's, savings accounts, pension funds, money under the mattress, everything. If there is real property involved; it must be appraised and assigned a value. From this monstrous exercise, the Medicaid office will then tell you what you will be allowed to keep and what must be liquidated / spent before Medicaid will provide any financial assistance. There are often financial limitations that outline as to the maximum amount of assets the Alzheimer's patient will be permitted to maintain at any given time. There could be a scenario that a provision is put into place that requires the individual to surrender a specific amount of money each month direct to a nursing home or a Qualified Income Trust and Medicaid pays the balance.

Walter retired from one of the local automotive assembly plants. He said he was taught to save, save, save all of his life so when getting to retirement, he and his wife could travel the country. On their first vacation trip following his retirement, they went to the Grand Canyon. Walter said he noticed that his wife was forgetting some of the details associated with their visit; small things like, did they have breakfast, and where are they going next. Details that would typically be in the forefront of her mind were missing to a degree. Since Walter worked 50+ hours a week prior to his retirement, his time with his wife was spent at the dinner table, in front of the television, or that drive to the grocery store and church. All familiar surroundings with little change occurring. Any memory issues just appeared to be very subtle and of no concern. This first trip was when Walter began to realize there is a problem. Upon returning home and losing his wife at a grocery store when she just wandered off, he decided a trip to the doctor was in order. It was then when Walter was informed that his wife has dementia and likely Alzheimer's Disease. Just over $650,000 later, Walter's wife passed and left him living in an apartment. He fell prey to changing tax laws at the time which left him with nothing.

Notes:

8. Join a Support Group

Have you ever had the experience of being in a strange area of town walking down a sidewalk where you were very uncomfortable with the surroundings? Across the street you see some older teenage boys roughing it up amongst themselves, ahead on your side you see a vagrant laying in the doorway of an out-of-business storefront, you see an older man with a trench coat approaching you and it appears he has something that could be a knife or a lead pipe in his hand somewhat concealed by his sleeve. His face looks to have somewhat of a chilling look to it. With each step, the two of you are rapidly coming to what can be a life-changing event. Your breathing becomes shallow. Then when this man is now less than five steps away his coat partly opens, you happen to notice something shiny, it is a cross hanging from his neck. What looked like a pipe is an umbrella and the look of death just turned into a huge smile and a heartwarming "Hello."

Through our lifetime, we often walk down these streets of the unknown only to find out that our fear was unfounded. Very much like dealing with a loved-one struggling with dementia. We do not know what lies ahead or what may lurk in the dark.

What can we do to protect ourselves from these difficulties? Well, for some, walking down that street surrounded by a dozen bodyguards may provide that needed comfort; most find other options. Some choose not to go down that street at all. If you have reached this point in this book, obviously you are not one of those either. Would walking down the street surrounded by those that can help and protect you from possible harm be something that would likely be the best option?

There are many sources for information where you can turn in order to obtain knowledge on dementia, the various medications, what to expect, its characteristics, the many life stories, and more. You have friends and relatives, the clergy, social workers, and care providers that can share information and administer comfort as well. When I was faced with the horrible dilemma of what to do next for my mom, a friend suggested a support group. I was quite skeptical. My thoughts were that this was a private matter. I wondered how these people could possibly understand what I was

You are not alone. Others are there to listen, share, and support you with your difficult daily challenges.

dealing with in my life. I did not want to go to listen

to other's problems when I was overwhelmed with my own. I am a guy, after all, I am supposed to be able to do this on my own! I was not sleeping, I had constant nausea, I felt like I was carrying the weight of the world on my shoulders and found myself going from severe anger to outbursts of tears within minutes. I thought about a counselor, but quickly realized that I am not broken, it is life that is trying to break me. Reluctantly, I gave the support group a try. What bad could come from one meeting? After all, it would give me an excuse that I felt justified to not have to be with my mom.

At my first meeting, I was greeted by about ten others and a facilitator. Not long thereafter came my time to talk. I was determined to get my story out in front of everyone. What I had not realized was how difficult it would be. Soon, though, one of the other group members handed me a tissue. The room was completely quiet while I struggled to share my troubles. Everyone listened intently, and no one interrupted. By the time the meeting was over and other members shared their recent experiences, I found some peace. These people knew exactly what I was dealing with. Some were living it, while others had become veterans. I found that I was not alone. These people were there to walk with me as I traveled down this street of despair. I received both information and comfort. Before long, these people became family to me. We all shared our experiences and brainstormed on ideas on how to deal with difficulties. The support group was the number one thing I did to help me make it through another day.

To be completely transparent, I also began listening to Elvis Presley gospel music. (Please don't judge me. It helped.) Eventually, I memorized every word from listening to his songs of inspiration. As I became more comfortable with my new group, one of the group facilitators announced his upcoming family move out of state. He asked me if I would like to take over his spot. I told him that I know nothing about helping anyone, not even myself, in dealing with the difficult dementia issues. He asked, "Do you know how to lead and manage a meeting?" I assured him that running meetings was a big part of my "day job." He said, "You are perfect, then." My mom was always so benevolent in helping other family members and with church activities that I thought that I will take the role as a tribute to her. I would never have thought how critical that decision was at the time. Due to her inspiration within me, I wrote this book.

Over the years, I have heard hundreds of stories. Not one of these stories was any less than another. Some members would attend on their own, while others would come with another family member or friend. There were those caring for a spouse, a parent, a grandparent, an aunt or uncle, a sibling, a child, and maybe just a friend. Their loved-ones were at home, living at a care facility, living on their own near-by or possibly across the country. These group members came from a multitude of occupations including a judge, an ER doctor, clergy, a few attorneys, an ex-congressman, some sales people, a few nurses, several general labor workers, the list goes on. **This disease does not care who you are or who your patient might be.** We are not given a choice as to whether we want to fall victim of this horrific path.

Soon after attending this group, I discovered that I was surrounded by some of the smartest people around. These folks around the room were all dealing with the same things I was dealing with and even had some answers to questions I was struggling with. Everyone was at a different spot along their journey, so the open discussion was helping everyone. No one dominates the meeting. A member shared, "One of our most important gifts is to share our personal story and experiences so we all can learn and benefit from each other." When a new member comes, some extra time is provided them, but overall it is truly an event that you begin looking forward to. My meeting met every-week, while some other local meetings were twice a month, or even once a month. I felt that the every-week format helped the members understand that we are there for them. Their questions or challenges do not have to wait for several weeks. People eventually develop a friendship with each other. Some even choose to become best friends. Certainly, the common denominator is the struggle they face in everyday life dealing with someone special that has become afflicted with dementia.

I had folks that would continue to come to the group even after their support member had passed. They felt that they can still help someone else with their struggles. The atmosphere was really hard to explain and something I have never witnessed anywhere else. There was no drama, no competition to one-up another, no arguing, no dislikes; just a group of people that loved the one they were providing for so much that this was where

This is far too big a struggle to handle on your own.

they found answers and understanding. **This is far too big a struggle to handle on your own.**

From a very high level, everyone was trying to help someone they cared about with the day-to-day strife of dementia. But at the ground level, there were no two stories the same. It was the team that would work through the issues at hand and come up with some answers. Even after being involved for over 20 years, there were still questions that would come along where even I had no answer. We would try to provide the best suggestions we could; sometimes the advice was very good and sometimes options were debated.

There are no written rules that would require someone to talk or share. At times, things get so tough that it can be very difficult to even speak without bursting into a pile of tears. (Not sure what a pile of tears is, but I have had them.) Even with new folks, I would give them the option to talk only if they felt up to it. It took me many months before I was able to freely discuss the difficulties my mother was experiencing.

An interesting outcome from this togetherness, sharing, caring was from an ER doctor. He attended in support of his wife in dealing with the issues she faced with her father. The doctor said that because of this group, he has learned some valuable information; information not learned in medical school or during his internship. He said that when a patient would enter his ER, it was all about a quick triage of the patient and begin administering appropriate treatment. He mentioned that his approach will be different. When treating a patient with dementia, he said, he may not know exactly what he might be facing. The patient may not be able to communicate effectively whether being verbal or physically capable. Touching a broken arm will cause most people to jerk or flinch. The Alzheimer's patient may not be able to express or even feel the pain. This doctor said that as part of his initial assessment, he and his ER staff will be including a cognitive evaluation as part of the initial triage.

Dealing with the unknown associated with dementia care is a real thing. Finding relief as a caregiver can come via different strategies.

1. <u>Ask for help</u>. Ask other family members, siblings, cousins, friends, and even professional hired aides. An aide is trained in working with the various daily life struggles you are experiencing with your loved-one.

2. <u>Embrace technology</u>. With rapid developments in electronic technology, our surroundings are getting "smarter." We can monitor and control video, temperature, security, living patterns, driving styles, reminders, alerts, music, and more. Medicine can be dispensed electronically at specific times and monitored remotely.

3. <u>Explore respite care</u>. Everyone needs a break. Sometimes we simply need to take time off.

4. <u>Review community programs</u>. Look around, you will find various resources that can be of help in keeping your loved-one involved. Whether it be the senior center or the library, it could be an adult day-care center or the VFW. Often your local county coordinators have information on these topics that they would love to share with you. Home delivery programs for food, personal items, and medical products are all possible.

5. <u>Share, share, share</u>. Connect with a support group or a therapist. Either can help you talk it out. We often find relief by simply getting it off our chest by sharing our difficulties with someone else.

9. Create a Respite Plan

You are absolutely no good as a care provider if you are not capable of helping. This disease will literally kick your butt so bad that your shoelaces will suffice as a necktie. In the care triangle that I referenced earlier, I mentioned that you are the most critical component of that triangle. Without you firing at full capacity, all the time, the level of care becomes something less. Eventually, as you wear down further, you will make mistakes, make bad decisions, and even forget. You will then begin believing that you have become the patient. Your health is more important than the health of the one you are caring for. Sounds heartless, I know, but it's a fact.

> **Most important rule for a caregiver: take a break. It is OK. It is not selfish.**

So how do you go about caring for yourself while caring 24/7 for someone else? I am glad you asked. Sometimes we have to sneak a break. Once you have managed to get your husband into bed or set up with his favorite television show, skip the urge to clean and instead, take a bath, or go outside and work in the flowerbed. Take a walk or just get into the car and turn on some music so loud it makes your ears bleed; so loud that you cannot think of anything else. Well maybe that is a bit extreme. You get my point. You can slip in a little respite time by going to a museum while pushing him around in a wheelchair. Go to the grocery and make him push the cart. Or, something most will not do, ask your son to come over to watch Dad while you go get a massage.

As this disease advances, your circle of friends will shrink. Your dinner at mom's house on Sunday will become filled with excuses. Let's face it, it is not much fun to sit and talk with someone who keeps repeating the same story, asks the same questions, or will simply not engage in the conversation. It is very sad to watch. Our visitors just don't know what to do or say. As a result, you begin to experience social anxieties. You start to feel all alone. You are trying to do your best to provide the care but feel that your life is collapsing all around you. You even begin to think that asking for help is imposing. You immediately assume that the other person will not want to help.

This is not something where you want to fail. What do you need for your survival plan to be a success? To what extent are you willing to go in order to maintain your health and your sanity? I will be upfront with you, most of you will not follow this advise I am about to share. Most of you are either too vain, too shy, too stubborn, too lazy, too controlling, too overwhelmed (do I need to continue?) to follow what I am about to suggest. Most of you will say, "Yeah, that is a good idea and I will do it tomorrow." Guess what? Tomorrow never comes! Tomorrow is just a unit of time that represents a part of the future. Tomorrow will never be today. I am hoping by reading this simple message, that you set this book down and immediately do what I am professing. Now memorize the phrase, "petere auxilium". In English, that is **ASK FOR HELP**. Right now, call four friends, family, clergy, co-workers, professional care provider companies; essentially, the first four names that pop into your head. Call them and say, "I need help!" For now, don't worry about where you need the help or how often you need the help or even why you need the help (that is obvious). Just ask, get their confirmation, and ask if your new help group can get together within the next couple of days to share ideas. Now why are you still reading? CALL! Please!

Did you call? Some of you are saying, I don't have any friends, or I don't have any family, or I am not a part of a church. I understand; we all have unique circumstances. Please allow me to suggest additional resources. Most communities have a community resource coordinator that should be able to share some contacts. Your local police or fire departments often encourage their staff to become more involved with community members; you just might be surprised. Many churches do not require you to be a member in order to receive volunteer services. Your local Alzheimer's Association is filled with a wealth of knowledge and contacts where you can find help. Please do not be the victim. I need you to be on your game. We will get past this together! Just as you do not know all the answers, your family, friends, and extended team know even less. Don't assume anything and certainly **don't assume no one is willing to help**.

Your first order of business with your new team is to listen to what and how they feel they can help. It could be doing the grocery shopping. It could be taking your loved-one for walks in the morning. It could be coming by and watching ballgames with your husband while you go to the hairdresser. It could be mowing the grass. It could be helping bathe your loved-one. There are literally hundreds of things where your team can be of help. It is now up to you to let them! If you start worrying how clean your house is when they come by or worry that your husband has not shaved for a few days before the visit, or even think for one minute that you "owe" them something for their help – I will tell you now, you will fail! This team is there to help YOU. It is YOU they love and want to see healthy. It is YOU that they care about and want to help. If your house is clean, grass mowed, husband shaved, and pantry stocked; tell me why they will want to help. Remember this, no matter what you do, there will never be more than 24-hours in a day. YOU need some of that time to maintain your health and your sanity. Let's allow 6-8 hours for sleep, 2-hours for personal care, and 3-hours for meals and prep. This leaves 11-hours for everything else, including doctor visits, sitting in traffic, and dealing with this incredible challenge facing you every day.

If you are a parent and feel you are imposing on your children, please remember, by nature, we feel better by helping others. Most children want to help their parents, at least in some form or fashion. I get it, you have things you do not either want them to know or culturally you feel it is not their business. All that is fine. However, you still need help and they are willing to do so. Grandchildren can also be a great resource for some of the "easier" tasks. Grass cutting or reading stories to Grandma are perfect ways where the grandchildren can be of help. Your children can help in more of the difficult tasks like managing the money, handling car or house repairs, and assisting with doctor visits. Why not start a new tradition and start going to their house, rather than yours, on Sunday for the "family dinner?" If Dad is too tired following the meal, you can leave. If he is engaged, you can stay for awhile.

There may come a time where sister Clare's daughter is getting married and you would like to travel out of state to attend the wedding. The trouble is that taking your husband will be very strenuous on him. Let's consider a few options. First, who can come into your home and stay with him while you are gone? For a trip of more than a few days, you can arrange for a second or third person to stay with him. The variety may be enjoyable for your husband. Second, there are facilities that provide respite care. I have seen some that will offer residency for up to 30-days. Normally, everything you need for your husband's care can be offered by one of these providers. Your community resource coordinator or the Alzheimer's Association can help you find a facility that should meet your needs. Section 3 in this book, will provide more detail on this topic.

I have worked within the engineering trades for many years. Did you know that the most dangerous building construction, from an earthquake perspective, is unreinforced brick or concrete block? I was quite surprised when I first learned this. Brick and concrete block can be destroyed by the shaking and moving of our earth's surface. Also, in seeing preparations that occur prior to the arrival of a hurricane, we see people boarding up their windows. Most think this is because of all the broken glass and allowing rain to enter. Actually, once the glass breaks, the internal structure of the building becomes pressurized to the strengths of the wind causing the structure to literally explode. Similar to the function of a parachute, it traps the air.

I use these two examples to demonstrate that the strongest of buildings give way to forces beyond their control. Changes to their construction is being implemented in order to strengthen their core. Just as with you, in order to keep your core strong, you have to reinvent and innovate. By asking for help, allowing yourself some time-off, and keeping healthy;

you will maintain a strong structure to best care for your loved-one.

Notes:

10. Assess Patient and Your Safety

A determining factor in deciding when to place a loved-one in a healthcare facility is determined via evaluation of the patient's environmental and physical safety. Face it, there are far too many "things" all around us that can cause us harm. As a healthy male, I cannot seem to be able to walk through a room without hitting my head on something. Consider if I were looking down while shuffling with each and every step; I would likely need a helmet in order to protect my head. (I should probably be wearing one now.) Regardless of living alone or with someone, the hazards can be fierce.

Environmental hazards – These are the various items we are exposed to that without caution can cause grave side effects. These include kitchen and cleaning chemicals, stoves, ovens, microwaves, blenders, mixers, garbage disposers, heaters, furnaces, air conditioners, fans, washer/dryers, refrigerators, freezers, irons, hairdryers, lawnmowers, weed-whackers, radios, televisions, hand tools, etc. For each of these items listed, I can list a half-dozen ways that someone can get seriously injured in using the device. Two common denominators from this list are chemical and electrical. All of these items are contained in most homes and/or a guest's home. As our loved-one progresses further into dementia, they will begin to forget how to operate or properly use these various items. They will begin confusing the purpose of the item and will associate it with a different purpose. For the most part though, the above list will not cause harm if used properly or simply not used. It is when the human factor comes into play that error can occur. It is when your loved-one tries to light the pilot light on an electric stove. It is when metal pans are put into the microwave to be used to heat water for tea. It is when someone reaches under the mower before the blade stops. It is when flour instead of baking soda is thrown upon a pan that has ignited on the stove. It is when the garbage disposal is making a noise and your loved-one forgets to turn it off before checking for the cause of the noise. It is when your loved-one turns the hot water on without adding some cold water and gets scalded. (A simple fix is to turn down the temperature on the water heater.) And, it is when the furnace is turned up all the way and you find your loved-one laying on the bed completely dehydrated.

These are all stories I know have occurred. I personally experienced the last one in caring for my mom. The fact is, it is not their fault that they cannot remember the proper and safe way of using a device or what to do in the event of an emergency. How many of us have gone out and bought a phone with bigger buttons or a remote control with bigger buttons in an effort to try to help your loved-one better use the device only to be upset that no matter how many times you instruct and re-instruct them on the use of it, they will still not use it correctly the next time.

Physical safety – These consist of accidents that occur due to the patient's inability to navigate whether moving, seeing, hearing, or eating. This category can include a fall in getting in or out of the tub, tripping on a throw rug, missing a step in the stairwell, not hearing the word "No," eating expired food, taking the wrong medication, grabbing something hot, not wearing sunscreen while outside, slipping on a wet floor at the store, dropping something that was too heavy to lift or hold onto, provoking someone into anger, and improper hygiene habits.

Most of these items are not specific to dementia and can or have happened to all of us. The challenge here is what happens next. Someone not experiencing any cognitive impairment can likely figure out what to do if he falls, eats something improper, causes a fight, or pulls a muscle in his back. A person with dementia is losing their ability to reason and likely in an aggravated weakened state. They may not be able to get back up or call for help. They may not have the ability to know how to get help.

Matt, a group member caring for his mom, said his mom complained that her neighbor would come into her apartment while his mom was out at the store and would steal something. She told Matt that it was money, clothing, and cooking items. Matt checked the door locks and discovered there were no deadbolts, just key-locks on the door knobs. She had two exterior doors and neither were very secure. Matt went to the hardware store and purchased deadbolt locks. Matt then had a friend stop by to help him install these new locks. Matt knew his problem with his mother's neighbor would be resolved. A week later, Matt returned to our meeting to report that his mom said her neighbor is coming into her apartment while she is out and is stealing things. Matt asked his mom how that would be possible. His mother said that the neighbor must have a key or knows how to "undo" the locks. It was then that we helped Matt understand that his mom may be suffering from paranoia. I asked Matt if there was proof that anything was stolen other than what his mom indicated. He said, "No."

There is an expression that travels through the Alzheimer's community that goes like this, "Never turn your back on an Alzheimer's patient and never get yourself trapped in a corner." Your patient may suddenly not recognize you and feel they need to take defensive action. Picture yourself in the kitchen getting a cup of coffee. You turnaround and there is a man standing there you don't recognize. At that point, you go into a fight or flight response. Protecting yourself is all you can think about regardless of what this man is trying to say to you. This is the same reaction your loved-one may experience with you. I strongly suggest the following:

- Remove all knives and other sharp items from vision within the kitchen. Out of site, out of mind. It would be best to reduce the amount of knifes and by doing so, begin keeping them in a different drawer than normal.
- Rid your home of guns. If you feel you need one for your own protection, I urge you to use trigger locks and gun safes. You should be the only one with access. <u>You need training in self-defense if you plan to keep a loaded weapon.</u> DO NOT TRY TO LOAD OR UNLOAD A GUN UNLESS YOU ARE

COMPLETELY FAMILIAR WITH THE GUN AND THE PROPER PROCEDURE ASSOCIATED. Your local police department would be happy to help with this matter.

- If personal security is necessary, there are chemical spray deterrents that can be as effective as a gun or knife. A gel spray is my choice in that it is very accurate and quite effective. It then gives you the needed time to summons help.

I know it can be a real challenge to clear your house of your husband's gun collection. After all, this is his castle and he feels a need to protect you and it. On the other hand, you may no longer be the queen of the castle in his eyes. Think about suggesting that the majority of the collection be in holding with your son and how honored the son would be to have the trust of his father in holding and protecting this collection.

The mother of my friend Tony was in a nursing home dealing with Alzheimer's. Tony's father decided he wanted to bring his wife home for the weekend. Upon getting her settled at home, his father knew how difficult it was for the rest of the family, combined

> Remember, your loved-one may not know who you are and may feel a need to protect himself.

with the never-ending pain he felt in seeing how the love of his life has nearly vanished; so his father took a bold step and decided to shoot the mother and then turn the gun on himself. This was a horrific tragedy for the family when discovered. The one part of the story that still lingered was that the mother survived the gunshot wound. Tony is still caring for his mother. So sad.

Following this occurrence, the family started reconstructing the pieces of the puzzle to where they soon figured out that their father was beginning to show signs of dementia as well. In the end, the pain was far more than the father could withstand. This was certainly an incident that simply was not foreseen. It was not the fault of the gun, nor anyone actually. However, it was just so heartbreaking.

An area where we do have more control but far too often wait until something bad occurs is with driving. An automobile is the one weapon that kills more people everyday than any other weapon. A message that came from a new group member, "Our dad has been diagnosed with dementia, and yes, he sometimes forgets which way to turn at an intersection, but Mom is there to help; so, what is the problem? This is his freedom, his right!" Likewise, others have freedoms and rights as well. The children in a fully-loaded school bus have freedoms and rights. That young mother with her 3-month old baby in the backseat, both have freedoms and rights as well. Whose freedoms and rights are more important? When is the right time to make that decision? Foolishly, I waited until my mother rear-ended another driver. Fortunately, the driver only received minor injuries. Let's not confuse freedoms and rights with privileges. Driving is a privilege.

As a dementia patient begins losing their ability to reason and shows signs of reduced mobility, their reaction times also become affected. Discerning between the brake and the accelerator is then a problem. Signaling in the wrong direction and/or turning from the wrong lane is common. Not being able to determine which way to turn or turn at all at the next intersection will cause weaving or braking that can cause other drivers to become affected. Sooner or later, if the keys are not taken from your loved-one, something will happen!

Is it easier to allow a car crash to occur than it is to take away the keys?

If your driver has been diagnosed with a cognitive impairment and causes physical harm to another person(s), there could become a potential personal liability lawsuit filed against your loved-one. In the

US, insurance companies are nearing a time where a proof of functionality test will be required in order to continue coverage. States are beginning to require drivers that have been diagnosed with a cognitive impairment to submit to driving tests every six months. Something to consider; your loved-one has been diagnosed with Alzheimer's Disease; he hits another vehicle causing a very serious injury to the other driver who is the primary income earner in his family and due to this accident will be bed-ridden for the rest of his life. The injured family hires an attorney that quickly learns that your spouse was diagnosed with a cognitive impairment. You chose to ignore the diagnosis and allow your spouse to continue to drive while knowing the possible consequences; after all it is his "right" to be allowed to drive. Now you be the judge overseeing this court case. This other driver is now no longer capable of supporting his family of four and will have significant medical expenses for the remaining part of his life; what amount of money should he be awarded. With a little luck, your insurance company pays out its maximum allowance, but now you are in a civil court. What amount of money is fair to award this man and his family? I am confident in saying that the court will not be favoring you at this time. You will likely be experiencing a significant lifestyle change almost immediately. And why? Because it is easier to allow an impaired driver to continue driving than to take away the keys.

Hopefully, by now, we are in agreement that we need to at least limit if not eliminate the driving. It is best to have a conversation sooner than later regarding driving. An agreement can be made, written, and reviewed that when the time comes, driving will cease. Those conditions include confusion on directions, last minute corrections, hitting the curb more than once in a week, and showing signs of excessive agitation toward other drivers. And why do I say sooner...your partner will be thinking more rationally and better understand the consequences associated with an accident more clearly.

If this time has passed, there are a few options I would suggest:

- Ask the doctor to write a prescription stating driving privileges are no longer valid.
- Ask the doctor to send a letter to the state requesting a mandatory driving examination.
- Hand a note to the evaluator at the Bureau of Motor Vehicles regarding the dementia and request he be not granted a renewal.

- Always be the first to grab the keys and state you will drive.
- Disable his vehicle. (Have a friend or mechanic help by removing some wiring under the hood. Getting a key made that will fit but not turn the ignition. Have a mechanic adjust the valve stem on the tire so it will be out of air the next morning).
- Send the car to the "mechanic" i.e. your son or sister to hide the car. Keep repeating that the mechanic is still working on the car.
- Put it on their heart to suggest donating the car to a family member in need or to a charity.

The most common accident that occurs at home with the elderly is a fall. A fall can occur from tripping, an ischemic attack (TIA), weakened navigation abilities, things left on the floor, getting up and walking too quickly, blurred vision, etc. You can see, from this brief list, how easily it can be for an older person with dementia to fall, therefore sustaining possible serious injuries. To compound these, let's not forget, we are also dealing with possible hallucinations, delusions, and disorientations.

I would like to suggest some ideas for helping provide a safer living environment for your loved-one while they are still living at home.

- Monitoring systems – Thanks to technology today, we can keep a watchful eye on our loved-one. Cameras can be installed, including a body camera. You can view the activity from another room, your office across town, or at your home in another state. If you see an unsafe condition, you can quickly react. You can call Dad and have him remove the hazard, call your sister and ask her to drop by and take corrective action, or in an extreme event, notify the medics or police. Monitoring systems can extend beyond cameras to devices that regulate temperatures, sense fluctuations in blood pressures, see who is at the front door, determine proper medication distribution, and track sleep conditions.

- Bathroom devices – Getting in and out of the bathtub becomes a very difficult task and is met with a very high degree of accidents. Rails installed around the bathroom and particularly in the bathtub, shower, and toilet area are nearly mandatory. There are tension poles

According to the CDC, in the U.S., an older adult dies every 20-minutes from a fall.

that go between the floor and ceiling that greatly assist in the transfer of the patient into or out of the tub. These poles have rotating handles that make the transfer much easier. Folks that experience trouble in navigation need something to help with their stability. By providing bathroom safety, it allows for continued freedom while also maintaining a level of privacy for a little longer.

- Child proof – Just as you have done with your children or grandchildren, you have to child-proof the house for your dementia patient. You will need to limit access to certain cabinets and drawers. Possibly locking the basement door to prevent your loved-one from entering unassisted. Adding a bell to the outside doors so you know when they are being opened. Remove sharp decorative items from areas in the event of a trip or fall. Imagine causing greater harm when falling on the little replica of the Empire State Building sitting on the coffee table. If your loved-one is living alone, you may consider disconnecting the stove/oven. Anti-scald devices added to faucets, including tub/shower will help avoid severe water burns. Ground-fault outlets installed are designed to prevent electrocution when dropping an electrical object into a sink or tub of water. Smoke detectors are imperative on every floor and in each bedroom. Keep floors free of ANYTHING that can cause a fall. In bathrooms, throw rugs and towels left on the floor are often unseen and therefore can cause nasty falls. Most surfaces in a bathroom are very hard. Proper fitting shoes help avoid slipping. All rooms, hallways, and stairwells should have a way of lighting the area before the patient enters the area. Bed height should allow for the patient to have their feet securely flat on the floor when sitting on the edge of the bed. Toilet paper holders need to be to the immediate side and not force the person to have to reach forward or turn around behind them. Towels should be easily accessible to dry hands without forcing your loved-one to reach beyond their comfort-zone. Place notes of instruction next to objects where there are safety concerns, such as thermostats, microwave, and washer/dryer.

A lifestyle change becomes necessary when considering the safety concerns of your loved-one. With modernizing the décor of the bedroom we now see a thicker mattress on top of the box springs which is then sitting upon a drawer set that rests on the floor. In my house, I have to start running from down the hallway in order to hurdle myself upward and upon the bed. In getting up in the morning, I find myself sliding down off the side of the bed like a sliding board at the local park; who knows where my pajamas went? Not very comfortable, I might add.

A final safety concern worth noting is the "roamers." A characteristic of Alzheimer's and a few other noted dementias is roaming or wandering. This characteristic is reported to be common, but within my small world, I have not seen that much of it. Regardless, this can develop and continue or be short-lived. You need to be prepared in the event it does become an issue. We tend to think that the wandering is because the patient is looking for something or someplace; or feels a need to check on something or someone. An ID bracelet is a very important tool to help your loved-one return home safely. Sewing an ID tag into their clothing is equally helpful. Be sure to notify your local police department if your loved-one is a wanderer. Keep an electronic photo of your loved-one easily accessible that can be shared with the police and media if your loved-one wanders off. Be extra mindful if your loved-one is still driving. You will need a descriptive explanation of the vehicle and electronic photo, as well. When possible, keep water and a blanket accessible within the vehicle. If you think your loved-one has left the house and you have quickly checked rooms and the outer perimeter, notify the police. The sooner a call can be made, the smaller the search zone will be.

11. Review Day Care

You have heard the expression, "I simply cannot buy a break!" Dealing with someone with dementia can be a full-time job. If there is something more than 24/7 then that is what this feels like. You get to where you have trouble catching your breath. Your loved-one can sleep, why can't you. Or, they sleep for two-hours and want to get up and roam around the house. Where do you find relief?

If you are not already aware of this option, please let me introduce it to you. It is called Day Care. Simply put, there are services that will take over the care of your loved-one for a period of time while you then can take a hot bath or go shopping or do some cleaning around the house. These services can be at your home or at their facility. They provide trained personnel that can engage your family member to best help in keeping them mentally and physically stimulated in order to best maintain that quality of life. Activities from games to stories, from music therapy to massage, and from movies to aerobics are all possible.

I believe most communities have a facility that specializes in the senior citizen. Some also focus on special areas such as dementia. These places are where your loved-one will find peers that likely have common interests. My mom said the only thing she found in common with everyone at the day care facility was that they were all crazy. At least she found something. You can look for titles such as Senior Care Center, Rec Center, Senior Resource Center, and Adult Day Services. They can be associated with a community recreation center, a medical facility, an Alzheimer's sponsored option, a religious establishment, a veteran-based program, or privately owned and operated. Fees are usually pretty reasonable, and some also provide for transportation and meals.

> *Adult day care provides mental and physical exercise for the loved-one; the caregiver gets some worry-free personal time.*

A good starting place is at your local Alzheimer's Association or the US Department of Health and Human Services. They can usually provide you with the various facilities in your area that best meet the needs of you and your loved-one. When talking with the facility, be sure to ask the following questions:

- What services do you offer at your facility?
- Do you specialize in dementia care?
- Is your staff certified dementia care providers?
- Is your facility licensed, bonded, insured?

- What is your staff-to-patient ratio?
- Do you have skilled nursing on staff?
- How is your food prepared and inspected?
- Do you provide assistance with eating?
- Does your facility provide for incontinence assistance?
- Is transportation assistance offered?
- How are contagious illnesses managed and reported?
- What type of activities are offered?
- How do you engage a patient that displays anti-social characteristics?
- What are your fees and hours?
- Are Medicare or Medicaid payments available?

Don't be too surprised if your loved-one does not want to go. Once you have identified a facility that fits your criteria, take your loved-one to visit the facility. Using the term day care may not go over well so try something different. You can use the rec center, the office, the activity center, the volunteer shelter, something you might know from their past that often they found interesting. Some have told their loved-one that they are needed to volunteer to help people struggling with memory issues. A fellow told me that his wife used to be a nurse. At the day care facility, she would walk around with a clip board and some paper and do her charting with all the folks there that day. It gave her a sense of importance and chance for my friend to catch a breath. Most will say that they do not want to go to this facility. At first, it feels like taking your child to kindergarten. However, in nearly all cases that I can recall, the loved-one finally adapted, and it became part of their routine. A woman once told me that her husband became so used to going to the "Rec Center" that one Saturday, he got up, performed his morning routine, and went down to the end of the driveway to wait on the facilities' bus. Unfortunately for him, the "Rec Center" was not open on weekends. This story is a great example of how routines can play a very helpful role.

To help break the ice at first, you can go there and stay with your loved-one. Maybe do some simple volunteer tasks for the first day or two, just to give your loved-one time to adapt to this new environment. By day three and four, you can ween your way out of there. In any regard, my advice to you is that you do not ask your loved-one what they thought of the facility. You will most likely get an, "I'm never going back!" Asking is like startling a sleeping baby or poking a very large bear. Either way, you will have to put on your combat gear and do something.   If the topic comes up, certainly respond, but do not start the conversation.   A positive comment like, "Did you see your friend Alex there today?" may help get you out of a jamb.   Eventually, you will find that routines always win.

Notes:

12. Visit Long-Term Care Facilities

"When is it time?" is a very common question I am asked. When is the right time to place your family member into a long-term care facility? Typically, I will answer, if you are thinking about it, then it is probably time to start. Unless you are very proactive and have subscribed to all the guidelines of this book; you are likely one that handles life as it comes. "I will worry about that when the time comes." One of my favorite expressions is, "It is great to have a tiger by the tail; as long as you know what to do next!"

This stage is the removal of the final freedoms. Many look to a nursing home or a long-term care facility as their final step before death. They think that this is where people go to die. I can spin these words to make them sound a little more glorious, but in essence, that is what it is. Sad to say. My mother said she never wanted to lose her memory and end up in a nursing home. Imagine the guilt that I then dealt with when I was left with no alternative.

From days of old, our long-term care facilities have improved radically. Certainly, there is still room for more improvement, but at least today, the focus is on Quality of Life. Most facilities know that they need to recognize their patients as customers and therefore treat their "customers" with respect and dignity. As the provider for your loved-one, it is your option to move your loved-one out of that facility at any time.

Remember, you are the boss, you are in charge. Stay proactive and do your due diligence in finding the best location that fits your given needs.

Let's define Long Term Care facility (Nursing Home or full-care). This is a facility that provides all the physical and medical care needs for an individual that is determined no longer capable of providing for themselves. This facility typically has a staff doctor, registered nurses, care-assistants, an activity director, and administrator. Skilled staff members are trained in various life sustaining techniques in order to provide for the full-care environment. In the US, Long Term Care facilities are considered a state-regulated entity. The state provides for inspections, dictates guidelines, and supports patient's rights. Some facilities are part of a larger company and may change ownership, names, and management from time to time. This section provides you with a checklist of how to choose a Long-Term Care facility.

As a caregiver, your two most difficult tasks will likely be taking away the driving privilege and placing your loved-one in a long-term care facility.

An Assisted Living facility may provide a similar level of care. By definition, Assisted Living is designed for those that do not need "nursing" care. The patient can usually provide for much of their own daily needs. The primary difference for the

Assisted Living facility is the lack of state oversight for patient's rights. The facility does not need to follow the guidelines that a skilled Long-Term Care facility must meet. The caveat here is that many of the Assisted Living facilities came to realize that they were losing customers to the Long-Term Care facilities. So, to remedy that, they began to hire registered nurses in order to upgrade their level of care and began suggesting that they can provide the same care as the skilled nursing facilities.

I am not going to recommend one type of facility over the other. I will leave that up to your judgement. I am only bringing you the facts as I know them to be.

In choosing a Long-Term Care facility for your loved-one, I have assembled some guidelines to use in helping with that assessment. This chart will help you determine what might be the best choice in finding a safe, comfortable place for your loved-one. Across the top of each column, you can identify five different facilities. Once you have chosen the best option or two, then you can go back, unannounced, and re-evaluate the same criteria. Use a rating of 1 = Very Poor to 5 = Very Good. Enter N/I for not important and an X for could not rate at this time.

	Long-Term Care Facility				
	1	2	3	4	5
Date:					
Basic Information					
The nursing home is Medicare-certified.					
The nursing home is Medicaid-certified.					
The nursing home has the level of care needed (e.g. skilled, custodial), and a bed is available.					
The nursing home has special services if needed in a separate unit (e.g. dementia, ventilator, or rehabilitation), and a bed is available.					
The nursing home has fully disclosed all costs associated with residency that includes medication, therapy, laundry, personal care, diapers,					

telephone/cable, etc.					
The nursing home is located close enough for friends and family to visit.					
Residents' Appearance					
Residents are clean, appropriately dressed for the season or time of day, and well groomed.					
Residents are sitting in hallways or in rooms, slumped over acting lethargic.					
Nursing Home Living Spaces					
The nursing home is free from overwhelming unpleasant odors.					
Are odors isolated to one area or generally noticeable?					
The nursing home appears clean and well-kept.					
The temperature in the					

nursing home is comfortable for residents.				
Noise levels in the dining room and other common areas are comfortable.				
Smoking is not allowed or may be restricted to certain areas of the nursing home.				
Furnishings are sturdy, yet comfortable and attractive.				
Staff				
The relationship between the staff and the residents appears to be warm, polite, and respectful.				
All staff wear name tags.				
Staff knock on the door before entering a resident's room and refer to residents by name.				
The nursing home offers a training and continuing education program for all staff.				
The guide can show you certifications on file for staff members.				

The nursing home does background checks on all staff.				
The guide on your tour knows the residents by name and is recognized by them.				
There is a full-time Registered Nurse (RN) in the nursing home at all times, other than the Administrator or Director of Nursing.				
The same team of nurses and Certified Nursing Assistants (CNAs) work with the same resident 4 to 5 days per week.				
CNAs work with a reasonable number of residents.				
CNAs are involved in care planning meetings.				
There is a full-time social worker on staff.				
There is a licensed doctor on staff. Is he or she there daily? Can he or she be reached at all times?				
The nursing home's				

management team has worked together for at least one year.					
Residents' Rooms					
Residents may have personal belongings and/or furniture in their rooms.					
Each resident has storage space (closet and drawers) in his or her room.					
Each resident has a window in his or her bedroom.					
Residents have access to a personal telephone and television.					
Residents have a choice of roommates.					
Water pitchers can be reached by residents.					
Floors are clean, corners are not collecting debris, walls appear recently painted.					
There are policies and procedures to protect resident's possessions.					

Hallways, Stairs, Lounges, and Bathrooms					
Exits are clearly marked.					
Hallways, lounges, stairs, and bathrooms are brightly lit.					
There are quiet areas where residents can visit with friends and family.					
The nursing home has smoke detectors and sprinklers.					
All common areas, resident rooms, and doorways are designed for wheelchair use.					
Bathrooms, showers, and sinks have no visible mold or soap scum build-up.					
There are handrails in the hallways and grab bars in the bathrooms.					
Menus and Food					
Residents have a choice of food items at each meal. (Ask if your favorite foods are					

served.)					
Nutritious snacks are available upon request.					
Residents are permitted to eat in their room if conditions warrant.					
Dining area tables include groups of residents conversing and eating.					
Staff helps residents eat and drink at mealtimes if help is needed.					
Activities					
Residents, including those who are unable to leave their rooms, may choose to take part in a variety of activities.					
The nursing home has outdoor areas for resident use and staff helps residents go outside.					
Facility has an activity director or coordinator on staff and publishes an activity calendar.					
The nursing home has an active volunteer					

program.					
Safety and Care					
The nursing home has an emergency evacuation plan and holds regular fire drills.					
Residents get preventive care, like a yearly flu shot, to help keep them healthy.					
Residents may still see their personal doctors.					
The nursing home has an arrangement with a nearby hospital for emergencies.					
The nursing home forwards critical information on the patient to the hospital upon transport and includes DNR, Living Will, and DPA.					
The nursing home has a staff member accompany a patient to the hospital and/or other care provider.					

Care plan meetings are held at times that are convenient for residents and family members to attend whenever possible.					
Facility prevents someone from entering the building without notification of staff.					
Facility offers monitored 24-hour access.					
Facility has a plan to notify family members when critical needs warrant.					
Facility has secured areas with very noticeable alarms that prevent patients from walking away.					
The nursing home has corrected all deficiencies (failure to meet one or more Federal or State requirements) on its last state inspection report and can share this with you.					

Additional Comments:					

"The Life Story" – Ward was a dear friend and older gentleman that I had the honor to meet through my support group. His wife recently passed, and he wanted to continue to attend the meetings. He had two reasons why he wanted to continue; one, Ward had a great interest in helping others, and two, this group became his extended family. I sometimes would refer to these folks as alumni. They have collected a significant amount of knowledge over the past months to years that they want to continue to attend in order to share and help the new attendees. These alumni members are also deeply interested in others in the group that have shared experiences along the way and are wishing to keep close.

Eventually, Ward was no longer able to drive due to his personal mobility issues. I began picking him up from his apartment and then taking him home following the meeting. We would talk about baseball, a bit about his children, a few items about his prior work-life before retirement, and occasionally, he would share some of his political or religious wisdom as well.

The time came for Ward to join his late wife in heaven. In reading his obituary, I learned that Ward had a Master's Degree in Electrical Engineering. This was a surprise because I understood him to be a retired firefighter from a local military base. As the obituary continued, I learned that he designed a few of the more elaborate power grids that serve some of our local communities. He was a charter member of his church and was on city counsel at one time. While working at his Electrical Engineering firm, he became a volunteer firefighter. Upon retirement, I guess from his first job, he accepted a role as a firefighter at the base. Prior to his second retirement, Ward became the Chief at the base fire department.

The Life Story provides powerful emotional, spiritual, and health benefits. This is an amazing tool to introduce you loved-ones to others.

I was so humbled in learning of his life story. What I believed to be a pretty simple, humble friend was actually a man that made a substantial contribution to his community, his family, and his career. He was a husband, father, grandparent, and a great grandparent. At Ward's funeral, I was overwhelmed to see the amount of people who came to pay their respect.

While in the nursing home, visiting my mother, I learned there was a fully tenured professor in the room immediately across the hall from her room. My mom was, of course, the best mom in the world, but outside of that, she had her own story as well. Her life story was not to the extent of my friend, Ward's, or the professor across the hall, but a pretty amazing story as well. Actually, my favorite one is one that has led me to you.

Taking the time to create a life-story for your loved-one can be very helpful in providing improved care for your loved-one. The many care providers at these various facilities are looking for common points of interest in order to help in their quality of life discussions. By including a life-story in with the medical charts, gives the medical professionals a better understanding of the patient. They may learn ways to redirect a conversation. They may learn of a common interest that will assist in developing patient trust. Also, they may learn of something that could help calm and comfort your loved-one.

Let's not think of a life-story as a biography. It is best to keep it to a length that is easily readable within a few minutes. Be sure to include interests and hobbies, work career or profession, achievements and accomplishments, educational specifics, favorite vacation spots, likes and dislikes, and favorite cars owned. Include family details like first name of kids and grandkids, cities lived, anything special or unique with regard to the family members, best friends' names whether alive or not, anniversary, honeymoon location, and favorite restaurant for family events. You can share some stories that you might recall that make your loved-one special. These could be a Purple Heart recipient; have climbed Mt. Everest; restored an antique car; performed in concert with the Rolling Stones; earned a Writers Guild award. Or it could be something very simple as sang in the church choir; would sit on the front porch and read stories to the neighborhood children; as a child would sell lemonade at the corner; or made a skateboard from an old ironing board and rode it down the middle of the street. I knew a guy that when he would shake your hand, he would always have a small Tootsie Roll candy that he would leave in your hand. It sure was not a big deal for him, but 30-years later, I still remember him.

Once you have put the life-story together, share it with friends and family. Ask for their input for edit or additions. Once complete, be sure to print it on a bright colored paper. This will help the document be more noticeable when buried amongst the stack of other documents inside the folder at the nurse's station. You can also frame the story and place it on the wall in your loved-one's room. Those visiting can also share in the most amazing life that your loved-one has lived.

Get started on this now. This is a great way to engage and interact by capturing old stories and memories together. I recall a trip to the ER with my mother one evening. Behind the curtain next to us was a member of my support group with her mom, Lilly. I listened to her mom verbally relive a time when Lilly was a young girl in her field playing with her horse, Dolly. Lilly would call Dolly and tell her mom to come and help her catch Dolly. I closed my eyes and could vividly picture her fun and laughter. What a beautiful story and memory. My mom said pointing to the drape, "That woman in there is crazy!" I smiled and felt blessed that I was the one that had the opportunity to hear about Dolly.

Notes:

13. Contact Hospice

All amazing stories come to an end. Just as with life, we reach a point when our body is ready to call it quits. We have given all we can and are ready for what is next.

There likely will come a time when one of your loved-one's care providers will ask you if you have conferred with Hospice. This is certainly the words we never want to hear; however, we do need to face reality. And, you will likely be surprised what Hospice can do for you and your loved-one. Let's better understand Hospice and how it plays a role in the quality of life setting for your loved-one. Hospice is defined as a concept that has evolved over the years into a philosophy of providing palliative care to a patient stricken with a life-ending illness. Restorative care, or curative care, that which we are most accustomed to, is designed to heal or cure us from ills or injuries. Palliative care focuses on pain management (not sedation), relief from symptoms and stress, combined with emotional and spiritual needs. Palliative care may also be offered outside of Hospice as a mechanism that provides supportive care while waiting for an outcome. This could be waiting on a decision (next steps) or maintaining a patient at a specific state or level of health. For the most part, Hospice organizations have expanded their scope from focusing on services related to an individual diagnosed with a terminal illness to also providing services to those with life-threatening illnesses. This expansion makes Hospice the preferred mechanism to help provide comfort to the patient and family members in the support of the final days and hours your family member has yet to share with us.

Some parts of the world refer to Hospice and palliative care in different ways. Hospice organizations, in the U.S., can be either non-profit or for-profit establishments. Where the money goes is truly not the point. What is important is the quality of care provided. A recent study shows that dementia patients daily costs are minimal compared to a cancer patient. For this reason, there has been a large increase in the for-profit Hospice organizations. However, it is important to note, the study also states that a for-profit organization is more likely to ask you to leave their program in the event that the patient becomes too costly to care for.

Hospice can provide a glorious end to a very long journey.
Alzheimer's is referred to as the "long goodbye."

It is important to interview your local Hospice organizations in order to make the best choice for your loved-one, you, and your budget. With that said, Medicare supports the Hospice process by paying a daily per diem. For some not-for profit choices, if there is no money, the program may still provide you with the needed care and support.

You will find services vary from one Hospice location to another. Some are full-service, meaning they have their own facility for in-patient care, they will come to your home, to the hospital, or secondary care facilities to provide whatever palliative care needs are required. Other Hospice company's will only provide home care, while others may provide in home and in a hospital/secondary care facility, but do not offer any services from within their own facility. Always verify that the staff are trained in dementia care. Hospice can be more than administering medicine and sponge baths. They may provide music therapy, counseling services including grief management, massage therapy, a Chaplain, medical equipment and supplies, speech therapy (for swallowing), 24/7 care, and sometimes a new friend to share stories.

You might say at this point, "I want this for me when my time comes!" I think that thought process is why so many of these Hospice organizations have come into being. They are looking to provide that dignity and respect your loved-one so needs in their final hours. It is truly an amazing program for the patient and the family effected.

"How do I sign up for this service?" Actually, it is easier than you think. Medicare requires the patient be certified as being terminally ill, or no longer benefits from curative treatment by a physician, and having a prognosis of 6-months or less if the illness runs its normal course. If once under the Hospice program, your loved-one outlives the 6-months, that is not a problem. However, it your loved-one begins to improve to where Hospice is not the best course of actions, you will be temporarily removed from the program. I have seen on several occasions where a patient will go on and off Hospice care and in one case that I recall; three times. An important fact; you can exit Hospice at any time and/or move to a different Hospice provider if you so choose.

Eventually, your loved-one will move on to their final place of rest. Through Hospice, until they are transported to their next place, sees to it that dignity and respect follows. As I am told, if your loved-one was a veteran of the US Armed Forces, their body will be draped with the flag. As for your ongoing emotional care, Hospice will continue to provide counseling services to you for your healing.

SECTION 3

Daily Tips and Tricks:

Here are some specific suggestions as to how to deal with the daily challenges you may face. I wish I could say these tips will solve all of your problems; wouldn't that be awesome? These are some techniques that have been tried and found to be successful. They will not work for everyone, but at least these give you some additional thought on how to solve your specific encounters.

Taking medicine...

"Mom, I need you to take your pills." Mom says, "What are all these pills for?" You reply, "These are for your heart, this is for your stress, and these two are for your memory." Mom barks back, "My memory? There is not a thing wrong with my memory!"

So, you now know this was not a good response on your part. "Remember"...Forget "Remember." Reminding her that she has a memory problem is typically not a good idea. Let's restate it like this: You reply, "These are for your heart, this is for your stress, and these are some vitamin pills the doctor wants you to take to help keep you strong." Mom says, "Okay. Thank you for taking care of me."

Mom may say, "Why do I have to take all these pills? I am not going to take them!" You say, "Mom, you are absolutely right. Take these now and I will call the doctor and give him a piece of my mind and tell him we think he has prescribed far too many pills." Mom says, "You will do that for me?" You respond, "Of course Mom, I love you." Mom takes her pills and you forget to call the doctor. If it comes back up, either repeat the same message or state you are waiting on a call back. (When you can do this fluidly, you will have mastered therapeutic fibbing.)

Calming your loved-one...

April shared a technique she uses with her husband that helps distract him from agitation and then begins to calm him. April purchased some videos that she can play on her phone. These videos are a vintage photo set played to a 50's music background. The photos are of cars, actors, athletes, household items, clothing apparel, and entertainment activities. It includes poodle skirts to rock and roll. April can play this video for him nearly anywhere. Similar videos can be found on YouTube. Louanne would play baseball games that she recorded on her DVR for her husband. He would be calm and entertained for an hour or so while she was able to catch-up on some household items. Louanne said that although the ball game was from a few weeks ago, her husband would watch them as if they were a live broadcast.

Doesn't want to bathe...

This is a very common challenge that Joanie was able to overcome. Joanie says that with her husband, he becomes afraid when he gets his face wet. Of course, when we take a shower, getting our hair and face wet is one of the first steps. Joanie has her husband stand (sometimes sit on the stool in the shower) and begins with his waist and downward. She washes his lower half and rinses the soap off of him. She then moves upward to his arms, chest, and back. Joanie washes his mid-section and rinses it as well. Joanie then has her husband sit on the stool and begins holding his neck in her left hand and tells him to look at her eyes. She smiles, tilts his head back gently, and slowly eases water onto his hair all while being careful not to get any onto his face. He continues to look into her eyes for comfort. She adds the shampoo and while still holding onto his neck with his head tilted backward, she slowly rinses his hair with the water. Joanie will then grab a towel and begin to pat-dry his hair. This will capture any water that might run down onto his face when she tilts his head upright. With a washcloth, Joanie will add soap and begin to slowly wash his face and ears. She then rinses out the washcloth and wipes the soap off his face and ears. This may require a second rinse and wipe. With the towel, she then dries his face. She then has him stand; with the shower hose, she rinses off his body from his neck down. Joanie says the trick here is two critical steps. One, wash from the feet to the top rather than our typical method; top to the feet. Second, she says is the eye contact, smile, and taking your time. This gives him comfort knowing that she will protect him. Joanie added that when recommending this technique to others, always be mindful of the patient's feelings.

Giving...

I frequently see where a dementia patient suddenly becomes benevolent. Their ability to understand the value of money may begin to degrade. In the example of Ryan, he said his dad keeps getting letters in the mail asking him to donate money or stating he just won a prize and to mail money in order to receive the prize. His dad then mails a check. Sometimes cash and sometimes uses his credit card number. Ryan is perplexed and did not know what to do.

It was suggested to have his father's mail redirected to Ryan's home. Otherwise, set-up a post office box at the local post office. Another suggestion was to limit the amount of money his dad would have available. A group member suggested writing down the father's credit number for the father's use, however, leave off a digit.

Won't eat...

This can be a result of a few factors. First, they may not "feel" hungry. This is a sensation, like pain, that is a common symptom of traumatic dementias. Some researchers tell us that as the dementia patient's pain threshold increases, their awareness of pain decreases. Others say that it is due to the persons inability to explain the sensation. This leads to a second factor; when we describe food items to our loved-one, it may be misinterpreted entirely. And, a third factor is a change in their actual taste of foods. A common interest is sweet foods. (Be sure to consult a physician if your patient is diabetic.) Adding a sweetening flavor to foods can cause a renewed interest in eating. We can't add ice cream to everything, but we can add a honey flavor. Other additives can be pineapple juice, coconut sugar and coconut cream, grated carrots and beets, orange and apple juice, caramelized onions, maple syrup, and stevia (derived from an herb). Some foods can be sweetened by adding a pinch of salt. Salt can enhance a food's natural sweetness. Just try to be creative. When all else fails, reverse the order of the meal. Try dessert first. Our taste buds are most sensitive with our first few bites. After a few bites of dessert, try some green beans, bites of chicken, or a meatball. A multi-vitamin could go a long way in offsetting a few lower quality meals. Remember, we are going for Quality of Life and not so much Quantity of Life. For more information on meal choices, you can consult a geriatric dietician or go on the internet for a variety of ideas.

Going to an event...

I get asked frequently about whether a caregiver should take his wife or dad to a family wedding or funeral. I suggest you review the following:

- Can your dad share a story regarding the person getting married?
- Is your wife's health to where she can be exposed to standing (or sitting in one place) for a long period of time?
- Can your wife be away from the bathroom for an extended period?
- Can/will your spouse engage in conversation with others?
- Do you believe your loved one will always be in a safe environment?

- Do you honestly believe your wife will have a good time?
- How will other family members or friends act in the presence of your dad? Will this be uncomfortable for you? Him? Them?
- Why are you going to this event? For her? For yourself? Or because you will feel guilty if you don't attend?

The two most important areas of concern are health and safety. When in crowds, we are exposed to many conditions that can affect our health. These conditions include airborne and contact infectious illnesses, limited access to the primary care physician, and possible loss of medications. When traveling, it is easy for us to get separated. If your loved-one is unfamiliar with her surroundings, it may surprise you as to where or what she might do. Waking up in an unfamiliar room may enhance confusion and agitation. Weather conditions are quite unpredictable at times causing delays, detours, and cancellations.

Think about why this event is important to you as the healthy caregiver. In my situation, family members were understanding as to why I did not want to bring my mom to her sister's funeral where services were a five-hour drive and required an overnight stay. By the time we would return home, she would have forgotten as to why we even made the trip. Final answer; ask yourself if the trip is for you or for your loved-one. I think we know the answer, so might I suggest reviewing the section on Respite Care.

Clinical trials...

As the medical industry struggles to find a cure to Alzheimer's, you may hear of organizations promoting "clinical trials". This is a process where a group of individuals volunteer to take a new medication while being monitored by medical professionals. This could be anything from a small yellow pill to a shot of Pure Agave Tequila (not really, but I wouldn't object to volunteering for that "trial".) This yellow pill could be a placebo or the real thing. The participant would take the pill as prescribed and the outcome is evaluated. There are also trials that involve life-change behaviors such as elimination of certain foods, aerosol sprays, cleaners, anti-perspirants, cookware, etc. Whether you receive the actual yellow pill, or the placebo is unknown to the volunteer. By volunteering for a clinical study, you are helping in the advancement of the elimination of

Alzheimer's. For your consideration, I offer the following:

- If your participant is taking the placebo, there will be no improvement and although it is necessary to evaluate in this manner, your loved-one's quality and quantity of life may be affected.
- If your volunteer is taking the actual pill, a side effect can occur that can snowball into other conditions. It is important to define in advance that if a side effect is discovered that your loved-one will be nursed back to health at no cost to you and for how long.
- Be sure your insurance provider allows for clinical trials.
- The trial can be time-consuming so be sure to obtain a clear understanding before you proceed with the final agreement.

If you are interested in participating in a clinical trial, I urge you to talk with your neurologist or the Alzheimer's Association to learn more about programs available in your area.

Please be patient...

At a restaurant, in the grocery store, or even at church, when our loved-one either tries to converse with or is expected to converse with another person that is unaware of their dementia, the assumption is made that everyone is on the same planet and can

> ## Please Be Patient
>
> **The person I am with has dementia and may need some extra time.**
>
> ***Thank you for understanding.***

equally understand the message provided. Of course, we already know that our loved-one may not be able to answer the unaware individual and therefore create awkward moments. This can lead to frustration on the part of both parties. It is for this purpose that I recommend you create a card similar to that here or obtain it from my website.

This card is also useful in the event your loved-one may present an awkward behavior toward children. Sometimes it is cute when a grandpa smiles and waves at a little girl two tables over, but when he continues to do this may cause the parents of the child to become upset. Or, when grandpa stops a child in the aisle in the grocery store and tries to start a conversation, the parent or a valiant servant may come to the child's rescue. Our changing world tells us that this may be a bit creepy. By handing the parents one of these cards, you can save everyone a great deal of confusion and awkwardness.

My husband ordered a mail-order pill that is advertised to cure Alzheimer's...

So, let's be perfectly clear, at the writing of this book, there is NO cure for Alzheimer's. There are drugs that are being prescribed that may slow the progression of the disease and some claim have stopped the progression. Also, there are drugs that are still in an experimentation phase (trials). As stated in Section 1, there are no two people alike. Markers within the human body will determine how a drug will function, including Vitamin D. If you recall, a low level of Vitamin D can negatively affect our immune system causing a possible acceleration of the dementia. Once a brain cell has died, anything associated with that brain cell is also gone. Although a particular memory is not stored on only one specific brain cell, that portion of that event associated with that brain cell is gone forever. This may explain why at times your loved-one may say something that you had thought had long passed from his memory.

A cure, meaning someone is already a victim of the disease, is not a reversal. Similar to a cloud in the sky; once it has passed, it will never return.

A neurologist shared with me that one of her patients ordered the Magic Pill for Alzheimer's via the internet. She forwarded the pill for analysis and did some further research on the pill's manufacturer. It was discovered the pill was manufactured in a guy's garage in South America and contained mainly calcium carbonate. The best this pill would do for this patient would help prevent heartburn. Unfortunately, this could also reduce the absorption of Vitamin B12, therefore, worsening the dementia. Please follow up with your doctor on any so-called cures.

Finding the right care provider...

This is referring to a hired professional coming into your home or independent living facility. Many think of this as a means to help the loved-one remain in his home longer. It is important to have someone that you and your loved-one can trust. It is said you can take months to years to build trust, but only one second to lose it. Your best source for finding a care provider is via referrals. Fellow support group members can share their experiences. Your local Alzheimer's Association can provide various agencies or individuals qualified to assist. The Area Agency on Aging can also offer advice. You will need to define what services are required, hours needed, and gender of care provider. The services will vary as to nursing care or personal assistance. The personal assistance can include bathing, light housekeeping, toileting, exercise, grocery shopping, laundry, medication, or just simple companionship. The gender choice is not discriminatory, it is the type of individual you and your loved-one (in particular, your loved-one) is comfortable with and can trust. Sometimes men prefer a middle-age woman, and some may prefer a younger woman. Men may choose to only be bathed by another man due to respect for his wife. Likewise, women may choose a middle-age woman rather than a man due to modesty. Outside considerations are the physical size of your loved-one, his dementia characteristics, and her openness to allow for a care provider. Be prepared to have a few false starts. Your service provider is used to the interview process and will be patient in supporting your needs. As a caregiver, **there is only so much we are capable of handling on our own.**

My mom is continually getting urinary tract infections – UTI's...

Rodney said his mom was constantly dealing with a UTI and just does not know how to help her. His mom has had a gambit of antibiotics which seem to make the UTI subside, but it comes right back a few days following her completion of the medication.

Needless to say, corrective action is imperative. Otherwise, other than exaggerated cognitive failures, conditions such as kidney infections, kidney disease, and various bloodstream infections due to the active bacteria can develop. When a UTI keeps resurfacing, this may be labeled a Recurrent UTI (sometimes referred as a chronic urinary tract infection.) Recent studies are saying that there may be an underlying bladder infection that goes untreated. Women are more susceptible to a UTI than are men. Although, when bowel incontinence occurs, the patient is at a much higher risk of developing a UTI.

Rodney did some individual research and began giving his mom a cranberry supplement and a probiotic. The cranberry inhibits the adhesion of E. coli bacteria to the bladder lining preventing growth of the bacteria. The probiotic places good bacteria into our ecosystems therefore strengthening our internal microorganisms. It is advised that you consult your urologist prior to starting with any alternative methods. As for Rodney, his mom has been UTI free for quite some time.

How do I deal with my husband's incontinence...

I applaud you for taking the initiative to show interest in this topic. You would be surprised by the number of caregivers that become completely overwhelmed in dealing with a loved-one's incontinence and are too embarrassed to openly discuss what they are experiencing. Our body is designed to intake liquids and solids that nourish and feed our internal systems. What is not needed must be eliminated.

At first, we think of these incidents as an accident. I suggest to you to begin learning from each accident. What transpired over the past several hours that led to this accident; was it food or drink, or was it activity related? You will learn what liquids pass through our systems faster that others. You will learn what foods are easier to manage than others. Keep in mind, everyone is different and how our body reacts to various liquids and foods will vary. Be sure to include his doctor for appropriate advice.

At some point, the accidents become systematic. It is important to avoid getting angry and shaming your loved-one. If you recall, there is a clinical disease involved here and your loved-one is not trying to bring you harm. Bladder incontinence is typically the first control issue. Believe me, this is significantly more embarrassing for your loved-one than it is for you. Start with a calm conversation, suggesting that the two of you are in this together and to not be embarrassed if an accident occurs. Ensure him that you are there to help. Suggesting more frequent trips to the bathroom and controlled intake of fluids can initially prevent most accidents. Covering furniture with bladder pads will safeguard the furniture and minimize urine odors. Introducing adult diapers will become the next challenge. This is another indication to them their illness is worsening. Instead of using the term "adult diapers", for men, use the term "protective briefs" or "disposable underwear." For women, try "fancy panties" or "disposable panties." I think we can all agree using the word "diapers" for adults is degrading. There are many types and sizes. I would suggest reading labels to be sure you are getting the proper type.

If you are caring for a parent, this process is extra difficult. No one thought they would ever have to look at Dad's junk. Yikes! So unless you are blessed with a support person that can do this task for you, keep in mind, you are only managing this mission because of the vast love you have for your Mom or Dad. It will be difficult for the first several times, but will become easier as time progresses. Tammi recommends wearing protective-disposable gloves, using disposable wipes, and acting with expedience. She says it seems less weird when it is done quickly and she wears gloves.

My father keeps getting annoying phone calls...

We live in a strange era. An era where scammers are so common that law enforcement cannot keep up. In particular, daily phone calls are occurring telling us that our computer is not working properly; or, the caller thanking us for last year's donation and can they count on us to donate again this year. Uh, sorry pal, I did not donate last year! It does not seem to matter as whether we have a landline or a cell phone, somehow, these scammers are finding us.

Tonya offered the suggestion of talking with the phone service provider to discuss "setting up selective call rejection and acceptance features". Many phone service providers offer some form of this service that either blocks or forwards unwanted callers, otherwise, permits wanted callers to ring through to the phone. This service will prevent the scammers from calling Dad, while allowing him to receive your call when you need to talk with him. Another option for the cell phone user is to forward all calls to voicemail and text Dad when you need to reach him. He can easily return your call with the push of a button. There are devices that can be added to a landline service that allows for remote control of the phone. Via an internet connection, a VOIP service can be added eliminating the need for the landline service, while still using the same phone that Mom has been using for years. The VOIP service can be accessed by a website remotely giving you, the caregiver, the ability to make modifications to the operations of the phone. You may find the VOIP option is less expensive than the traditional landline option. Another plus to consider when moving to the VOIP is your option to keep the existing phone number or get a new one.

How often should I go visit my husband at his long-term care facility...

You should visit as often as you feel the need. Let's expand on this a bit. There are several reasons for visiting your loved-one in his long-term care facility. Of course, the first and primary reason to visit him is due to your unending love you have for him. As couples age, it is fascinating to see how their love for each other continues to grow as well. A second reason for visiting is to ensure he is getting the proper care and the facility's standards meet yours. You will see other visitors helping in the feeding, assisting in exercise, participating in activities, and taking a role in the personal needs for the loved-one. By keeping a visible presence at the facility, it will often cause staff to take notice and therefore be sure the quality of service they provide will meet or exceed your expectations. I would like to add that you visit at different times of the day to not be predictable. A third reason for visiting that many have shared, is to maintain the feeling of companionship the two of you have shared for so many years. And, the fourth reason is to meet with other caregivers there visiting with their own loved-ones. Creating this extended friendship will help offset the difficulty experienced in watching the change occur with your loved-one. By having another person to share your concerns helps in the healing; much like the values of a support group.

Due to the emotional challenges you experience in visiting with your loved-one, may indicate you should not visit as often. I mentioned earlier in this book, when I would leave from visiting my mom, I would sit in the car crying, uncontrollably at times. As dementia continues to take its toll, you may find your loved-one does not remember you did not visit with him yesterday. Time eventually becomes irrelevant. You could walk out of his room for ten-minutes, return and be greeted like this is a new visit.

When your loved-one is first placed in the long-term care facility, you may be asked by the staff to not visit for a week or so in order for your husband to adapt to his new surroundings. The greatest difficulty usually occurs within the first few days. Your intervention could prolong his adoption timeframe. Following this initial period, it is completely up to your own discretion as to how often and for how long you should visit.

How can I know if these various drugs are not causing an unpleasant side-effect...

There are times where multiple medications, foods, and supplements when combined can cause unpleasant side-effects. The side-effects can be displayed in various forms and can include a rash, an anxiety disorder, reduced cognitive abilities, a lethargic condition, or physical bodily function change. There is a medical professional that often can help in identifying side-effects associated with medications and that is a pharmacist. The pharmacist often maintains a Doctor of Pharmacy degree and is educated in human anatomy, organic chemistry, pharmacology, immunizations, and oncology; to name a few. By talking with your pharmacist, it may be possible to determine if there is a drug interaction causing a specific side-effect. If you are getting your prescriptions filled via their pharmacy, the feedback from the pharmacist is likely free. Although, the pharmacist cannot prescribe a change in medicine, they can contact your physician or at least advise you to talk with your physician regarding a change in medication that might reduce or eliminate the side-effect.

In closing, it has been truly an honor to have been able to share these words with you. I am hopeful you found benefit and will now be more empowered to take on another day.

References

Alzheimer's Hot Line (24-hour) USA........ 800-272-3900

Alzheimer's Web Information .... www.alz.org

Lewy Body Dementia Assoc. 800-539-9767

Lewy Body Dementia LBDA .... www.lbda.org

Agency on Aging www.n4a.org

American Council on Agency.......
www.medicaidplanningassistance.org
(Medicaid Planning Assistance)

Congressperson locator ....
www.whoismyrepresentative.com

Veterans Affairs .... www.va.gov

Medicare .... www.medicare.gov

Medicaid .... www.medicaid.gov

Epilog

I am often asked if I had a family member affected by dementia as to the reason for writing this book. My response is, "Yes, my mother had Vascular Dementia, but that's not the only reason for writing this book." In sitting through support group meetings, literally over 700 meetings, I learned a lot about dementia care. I also, met hundreds and possibly over a thousand people dealing with a loved-one robbed of his or her memory by these horrible traumatic diseases. I was raised in a Christian home, surrounded by Christian parents. My dad was a lay-minister, elder, trustee, and Sunday School teacher. My mother was a deacon and active in the women's ministry. I cannot recall not being part of a church in some capacity. I learned some very valuable Christian values as I traveled through my life. A specific value that I would like to share is in helping others without expecting anything in return. In seeing how millions of people are struggling mentally, physically, and spiritually with the impact that Alzheimer's and the like has upon their lives, I became inspired to do more than just lead a support group. I chose to write a book that would help caregivers. When I first got started, I was about 25%

into my writing when I mentioned to someone about my book. I mentioned that my goal is to put a text book into a caregiver's hand that will empower him or her to at least face another day. I said my goal was not to expect anything in return. I was told, "Oh no, what you are doing is Oprah stuff. This book can make you a lot of money!" It was then that I ran into writers-block. I could barely form a sentence. It was almost ten-years later when, I believe, God told me, "There is something I need you to complete." Was it projects at home? (I am a guy; there are always projects left undone.) Was it projects at church? I began my pursuit to complete tasks at home and at church. Again, I got the same message from God, "There is something I need you to complete." This prompted me to ask God if He can be more specific. I said that I will be obedient and do as You ask. I got no response and continued with my tasks. Finally, seeing an end to my projects, I asked God again, "Can you please open a door, throw me on the ground, slam my hand in a drawer; please tell me what it is that you want me to complete." The message came back, "Book." The book? Why does God want me to complete the book? A few days later, I asked again. This message was, "Book, book, book!" I could not even interrupt God's words. It came across loud and clear. In talking with my wife, I asked her why she thought this book was so important to God. She said it was likely because it is designed to help so many people; God's people. My writing resumed and became so fluid. I was writing about topics where the words just kept coming to me. It was like I was just moving my fingers on the keyboard to the letters where my fingers were being touched. As to why I stopped writing before, I came to realize that I was writing it for personal gain and not for God's glory. I got distracted in my writing more recently, but know who is doing the distracting. The very one that does not want to see people helped. The one that does not want to see God glorified. For this reason, my wife and I have labeled this book, God's Book.

NOTES:

NOTES:

NOTES:

NOTES:

12867308R00131

Made in the USA
San Bernardino, CA
12 December 2018